HOW TO
LIVE LIKE A
CRAZY RICH
ASIAN

HOW TO LIVE LIKE A CRAZY RICH ASIAN

THE ULTIMATE GUIDE TO THE FASHION, FOOD, PARTIES, AND LIFESTYLE OF SINGAPORE

Philip Choo

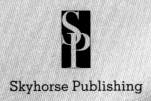

Skyhorse Publishing

Skyhorse Publishing books may be purchased in bulk at special discounts for sales promotion, corporate gifts, fund-raising, or educational purposes. Special editions can also be created to specifications. For details, contact the Special Sales Department, Skyhorse Publishing, 307 West 36th Street, 11th Floor, New York, NY 10018 or info@skyhorsepublishing.com.

Skyhorse® and Skyhorse Publishing® are registered trademarks of Skyhorse Publishing, Inc.®, a Delaware corporation.

Visit our website at www.skyhorsepublishing.com.

10 9 8 7 6 5 4 3 2 1

Library of Congress Control Number:2019945261

Cover design by Brian Peterson
Cover photo: Getty Images

Print ISBN: 978-1-5107-4683-1
Ebook ISBN: 978-1-5107-4684-8

Printed in China

For my mom and dad.

CONTENTS

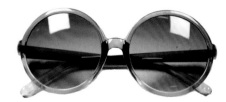

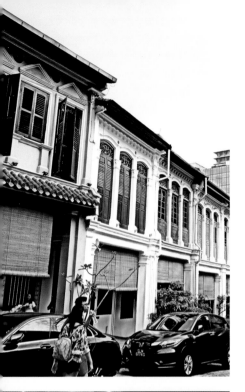

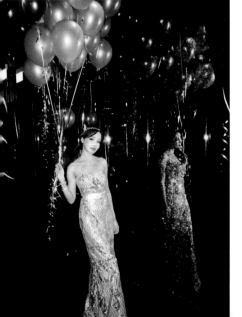

INTRODUCTION

"Nice to see you again, Emily, are you still staying on Emerald Hill?" I asked casually after taking my seat at a friend's wedding.

"Actually, my grandfather passed away recently and my family sold the home to a young couple a few weeks ago," came her reply.

"No way! My friends in their thirties just bought a home on Emerald Hill!"

As it turned out, Singapore really is that small—one of my friend's homes was sold to another friend of mine.

In our sunny city-state of 5.6 million people, it is extremely easy to find common friends and you can easily find connections when discussing school and workplace. Everything from idle gossip to scandals are spread like wildfire once the doors are shut and the backs turned. Like one of the first scenes featured in the movie *Crazy Rich Asians*, when the news of Nick's decision to bring Rachel to Singapore reached his

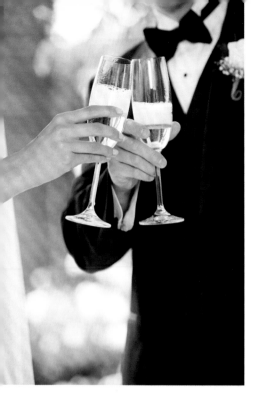

mother in two minutes, news is spread very easily, which can make it fun and exciting to live here.

On the surface, everyone keeps a poker face and doesn't intrude even if they see a celebrity. It's our culture to be a little reserved and not make a big deal about anything. Sometimes when you see an acquaintance on the streets, you might even walk the other way because you just hugged and said hello two days ago and have run out of lame greetings! People are sometimes not that warm, but the weather is really warm, all year round. However, if you got slapped in public or if you slept with someone new, you can be sure *everyone*—and I mean everyone—will know about it.

In the next few chapters, I will be sharing some juicy gossip and also the top places to go, and the things to eat or buy in order to channel your inner Crazy Rich Asian. Driving top down in a Ferrari and shaking your Richard Mille watch in peoples' faces is cliché and not that classy. Over here, the real Crazy Rich Asians have a fabulous lifestyle but may drive a regular Japanese car out of their palace like Astrid. Like how Nick Young says that they are just comfortable—but are actually filthy rich.

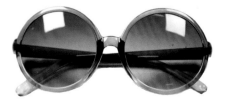

CHAPTER 1:
WEDDINGS

SAY "I DO" IN STYLE!

A wedding is one of the most important events of a person's life, and every couple wants theirs to be perfect. There are many who will go to great length to make their weddings memorable—sometimes crazy and crass, sometimes ostentatious, and sometimes just pure magical.

There are weddings in Singapore that are like a never-ending commercial, with everything sponsored and the magic forced. There are also weddings that are dramatic and theatrical, with every family member singing from every corner of the ballroom and the bride and groom putting on a show, high in entertainment with everyone laughing with you—or maybe, at you. Sometimes, class is something money cannot buy.

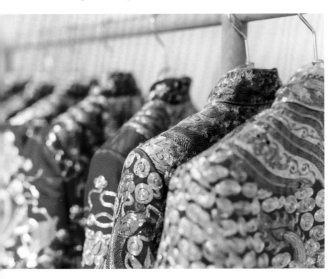
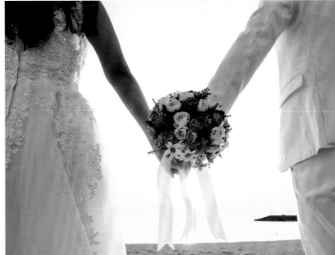

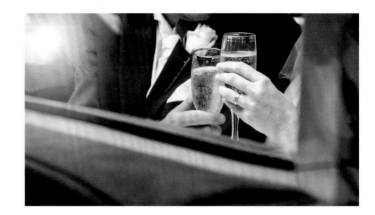

The ideal wedding is stylish and sophisticated without being stiff, heart-warming and fun without being overly dramatic. Though perfection is a relentless pursuit, the two weddings featured here come very close.

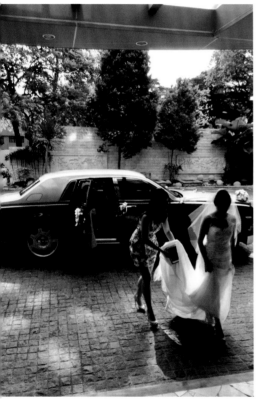

A Chinese wedding in Singapore is usually a full day affair, with "gate-crashing" being the first order of the day. The groom with his groomsmen will go through several stages of "obstacles" (some may call it torture) designed by the Angpow-hungry bridesmaids before he can win the bride's hand in marriage (bridesmaids usually allow the groom and groomsmen to advance in the various stages of torture when they receive a handsome sum of money found in red packets called Angpow). Having deep pockets will make the life of the groom a lot easier. Obstacles could include body contortion into various shapes according to the bridesmaids' desire, drinking concoctions that are sweet, sour, bitter, and spicy, meant to represent married life and getting through good and bad times together, doing a crazy dance, and on the extreme end, shaving your legs and armpits, or even eating worms.

This will be followed by a tea ceremony, where heirlooms and blessings will be showered upon the bride and groom after they serve tea to their family. Depending on the religion of the families, a church wedding in the morning or afternoon could also be included. After the affairs in the morning and afternoon, the couple will proceed to the dinner venue for a lavish banquet dinner where their distinguished guests will attend and join in the celebrations.

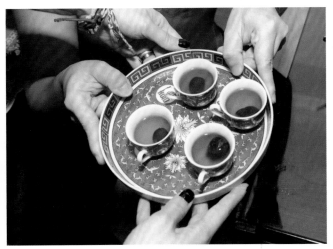
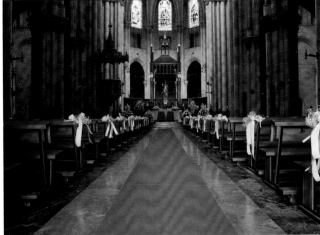

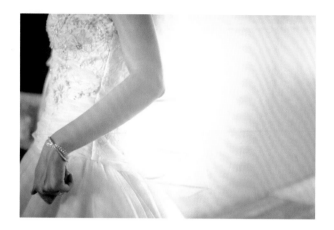

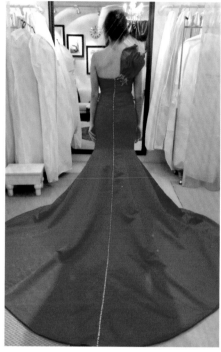

The bride rarely gets a chance to eat during the entire night because first of all, she has to fit into her very form-fitting gowns, and secondly, she has to go through at least three outfit changes and two march-ins at the dinner. Wedding banquets in Singapore are rarely held outdoors like the one featured in *Crazy Rich Asians* at Gardens by the Bay because our weather is extremely humid and wet, with periodic showers all the time. To put it simply, it is gross to be dressed to the nines and brave the outdoor heat! You can be sure that all your guests will be complaining and standing by the fans and not caring about your wedding speech if the event is outdoors without an air-conditioned tent.

This is why hotels are top choices for weddings in Singapore and prices for a table can be crazy. At five-star hotels, rates are usually between SGD $180 to $350 per person (about USD $130 to $250)—usually for food alone. A usual wedding size in Singapore is around two to three hundred people and for established families, anything from five hundred to a thousand people is possible. As Chinese people are very practical, giving Angpows (red packet with money) is the social standard for "blessing" the couple, and is much preferred over giving wedding gifts. Each year, a search online will have the latest updated list on how much is appropriate to give when attending a wedding at a particular hotel. The Angpow guideline even breaks down the price to weekend or weekday rate and whether it is a day or nighttime wedding. You can always give more than the recommended rate if you really love the couple. Everyone is expected to write their names on the red packet—giving less is frowned upon, so if you do, it may be the last time you will be seeing the couple.

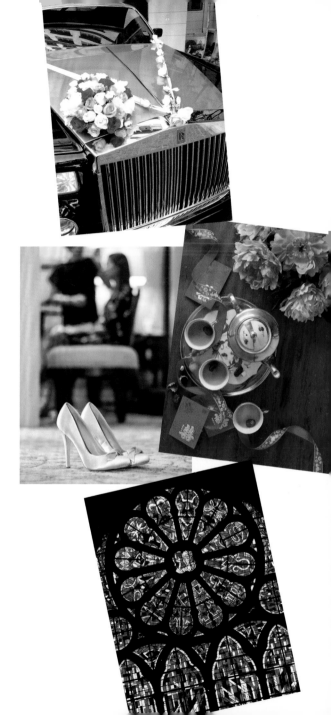

THE WEDDING OF RACHEL AND PO LOONG

On the rooftop of a sea-facing villa in Bali, Rachel said "yes" to her soon-to-be husband Po Loong who planned a surprise proposal while on a vacation with their closest friends. When choosing a wedding venue in Singapore, the couple wanted the same relaxed vibe near the sea and W Singapore at Sentosa Cove was the perfect choice. Some other conditions for the wedding venue were that it needed to be able to fit around five hundred people and that the food had to be amazing since Po Loong is a restauranteur in Brunei.

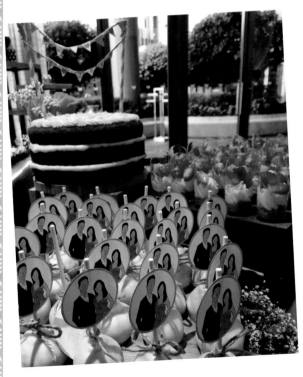

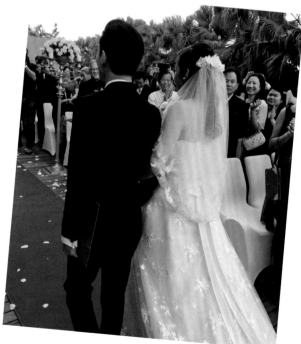

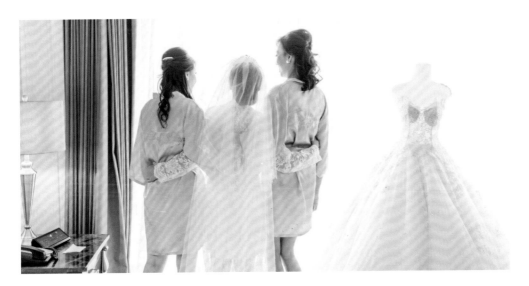

Having known each other for more than fifteen years since their college days in Canada, Rachel and Po Loong said their vows on a deck facing the Marina at sunset with their closest friends and family, all of whom have witnessed their journey together right from day one. After the intimate ceremony, they changed into a different gown and suit to greet the arriving guests—both of which had been designed by Singaporean celebrity bridal designer Michelle HuiMin. Bridesmaids' dresses were designed by Rachel's good friend, Evon Tan, a local designer based in Melbourne.

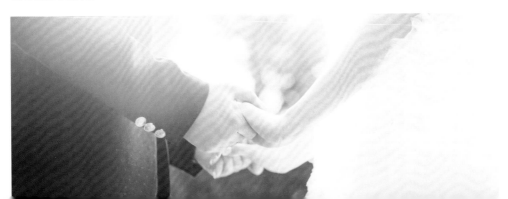

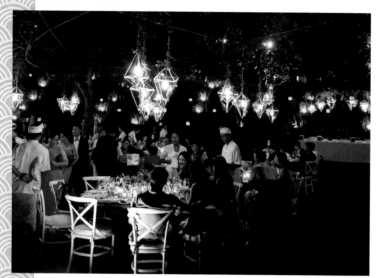

The night ended on a high when everyone raised their glasses to shout out the traditional "Yum Seng!" a traditional Singaporean toast done three times with the words belted out at the top of everyone's lungs. The louder it is, the greater the blessings for the couple to have a blissful married life.

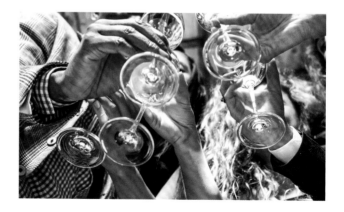

The Wedding of the Decade

In true CRA fashion, the original wedding we were going to feature was pulled at the last minute after the couple's parents objected to their wedding photos being published in our book. Like the character Astrid, they do not desire unwanted attention and we respect their decision. Below is the story of Lynette and Alwin (name and photos have been changed, of course).

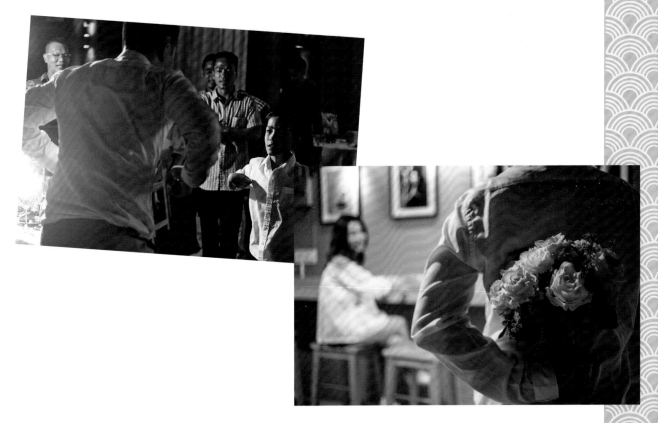

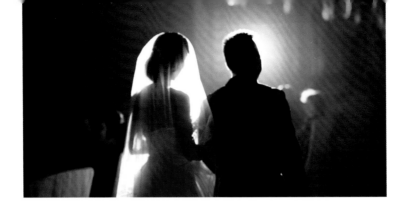

Having met in Junior College when they were seventeen years old, Lynette and Alwin's teenage love story has blossomed into a fairytale wedding that saw the attendance of some of the most important people in Singapore. The wedding day started with the gate-crashing ceremony when the groom had to go through "obstacles" to win the hands of the bride. The groomsmen arrived in a fleet of adorable Mini Coopers led by a vintage Rolls-Royce bridal car. They were greeted by a group of beautiful bridesmaids dressed in rainbow colors and armed with "torture" ideas to test Alwin's love for Lynnette. This was followed by a rainbow-themed church wedding at CHIJMES, where the bride and groom with their entourage had a joyride with a fleet of traditional trishaws—three-wheeled passenger carts which were used as taxis in the past. CHIJMES is the very same venue featured in *Crazy Rich Asians*, though this wedding was a few years prior.

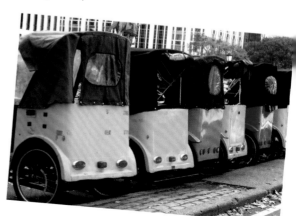

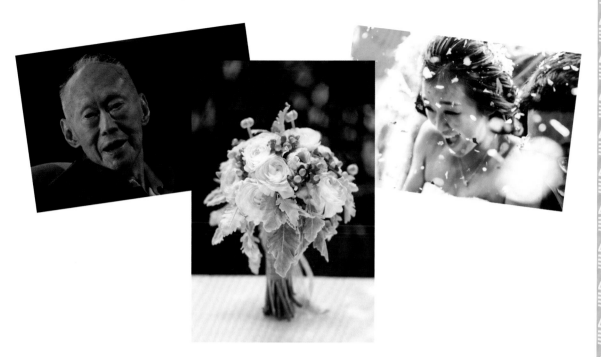

In the evening at Shangri-La Hotel's grand Island Ballroom, distinguished guests were treated to a lavish affair. There was an extra sense of excitement in the air because the founding father of the country, Singapore's first Prime Minister, Mr. Lee Kuan Yew, was gracing the event. Together with him at the wedding was the current Prime Minister Mr. Lee Hsien Loong, former Prime Minister Mr. Goh Chok Tong, and former Presidents Mr. S. R. Nathan and Dr. Tony Tan. The ballroom was beautifully decorated with lush white blooms, which guests were welcomed to take home after the event. The wedding had a white theme and the flowers in vases of varying heights transformed the ballroom to feel like a rainforest canopy. Lynnette wore a gorgeous gown by Monique Lhuillier and it was a night to remember for many, being in the same room with all of the country's most important people.

Crazy Rich Fact: China Wine

A famously charismatic Singaporean church by the name of City Harvest was in the news for all the wrong reasons. Founded in 1989 by Pastor Kong Hee and his pastor-turned-pop-singer wife Sun Ho, the church has grown in popularity over the years and is estimated to have a following of at least thirty thousand members in Singapore and other countries. Well known to many for its chic image and wealth-focused style of Christianity, the church had plans to launch a pop-singing career for Sun Ho in Asia and the United States by misappropriating the church's funds.

Launched in 2002, the Crossover Project was a scheme by the church to begin Sun Ho's pop-singing career and to establish her as a "demure singing pastor" in Asia. Her Mandarin singing career was hugely successful as Sun Ho topped the charts and held record sales after being marketed as a refreshing, warm, and loving pastor pop singer. Or so we thought. It was later reported that the church members had to fork over SGD $500,000 (USD $360,000) to purchase 32,500 of her unsold Mandarin albums—for losses of almost $1 million.

After the perceived success in Asia, City Harvest soon looked to the United States for a chance at cracking the global market. Sun Ho tried to shake off her pastor-singer image in favor of becoming a dance music singer (with the hopes of becoming an Asian version of J. Lo). She had a major image makeover in 2007 and threw her demure look out the window. Adopting a new nickname—"Geisha"—Sun Ho's new music video "China Wine" had her prancing around and twirling her hair in a tiny, barely there leather shorts and crop top, all in hopes of spreading the word of God through her music. In the video, she played the role of an exotic Chinese dancer and her follow up single "Mr. Bill" had her singing about murdering her husband. This was to little success, but raised many eyebrows back home in Singapore. Her lavish lifestyle in Los Angeles, which included living in an expensive Hollywood Hills mansion, also got many talking.

Pastor Kong Hee, Sun Ho's husband, touted her as the next Whitney Houston. He made everyone in the church believe that she was going to be a huge success and preached the possibility of her selling millions of albums and becoming the next big singing sensation. A shell company called Xtron, a music production firm, was set up to misuse the church's funds for this purpose. In the end, a total of SGD $50 million (USD $36 million) was dedicated to the Crossover Project, SGD $24 million (USD $17 million) to fund her singing career, and another SGD $26 million (USD $19 million) to cover up the scandal before the authorities came knocking.

Some of the church's efforts to groom Sun Ho into a global superstar include hiring famous American producer Wyclef Jean to help produce her record. He was reported to have been paid USD $1.5 million. Missy Elliott, a famous rap artist in the United States, had an appearance in her video to boost her street cred, and was paid USD $1.5 million as well. Even veteran record producer and sixteen-time Grammy Award winner David Foster was roped in to produce her debut English single, "Where Did Love Go." The song did, however, reach the top spot of *Billboard*'s dance breakout chart. How a single gets to number one is based on reports of a select few influential DJs playing the tracks and judging the audience's response, and does not necessarily translate to commercial success.

Sun Ho's career came to a crashing end in 2012 when her pastor husband and five other senior City Harvest Church members were arrested. They were put on trial and found guilty, ending her hope of any last shot at stardom. The leaders of the church, however, remain firm that they have done no wrong despite all the evidence. All they had were sincere and honest intentions in doing God's work and their church members agree and continue to give them their full support. But all Singaporeans had for them was scorn and criticism. Sun Ho, who was found to be not involved in any of the wrongdoings, said that the church leaders had "placed their faith in God and trust that whatever the outcome, He will use it for our good."

Preaching of the "prosperity gospel" is the draw of City Harvest Church. The church takes its inspiration from other charismatic churches in the United States and has great appeal to the middle and working classes in Asia. Its super cool pop concert–like services housed in a church made of titanium has fashionably dressed pastors and worship leaders luring young adults with free donuts and coffee after services.

By linking wealth to Christianity, the idea is that the stronger the faith and the more money one gives to the church, the more wealth one will eventually get back from God. It is an enticing message for many and City Harvest celebrates monetary sacrifices made by church members. By being sensitive to capitalism and consumerism, City Harvest has made the church-going experience very relevant to the real world in the eyes of its congregation and at the same time offering them a sense of community.

Despite Pastor Kong Hee and the senior members serving their time in jail, Sun Ho remains a star in the hearts of her church members. Leadership in charismatic churches like City Harvest is more personality-based and is less reliant on structures within the institution. The scandal has not dimmed the lights for Sun Ho in her church, and she is set to lead the church to greatness while her husband gets a chance at preaching to his fellow inmates.

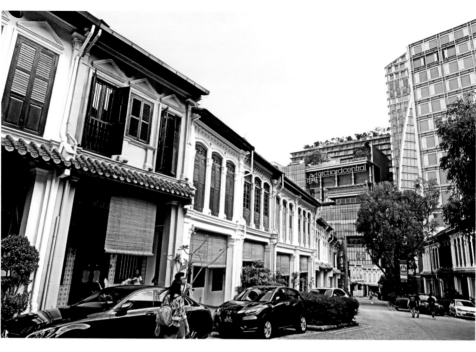

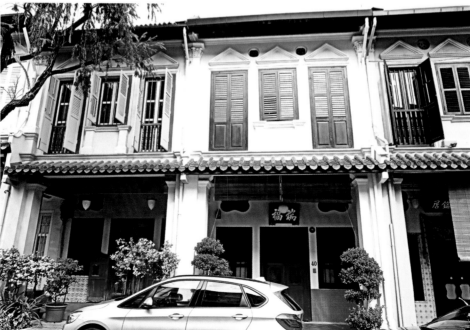

CHAPTER 2:
HOMES & NEIGHBORHOODS

Goh Peik Lin's Home

Nestled in a lush neighborhood by the Botanic Gardens, the family home of Goh Peik Lin used in *Crazy Rich Asians* is one of the hottest locations for die-hard fans of the movie and book series. This is an area in Singapore housing the top 1 percent of the country's elites. Back in June 2017 when the production of the movie came to Singapore, the home was in the market for rent and the look and design of the house suited the character's family perfectly. It's gold and the baroque-inspired facade was a great fit as the character Goh Peik Lin in the book rolls up to pick Rachel up in a gold BMW and wore golden sandals.

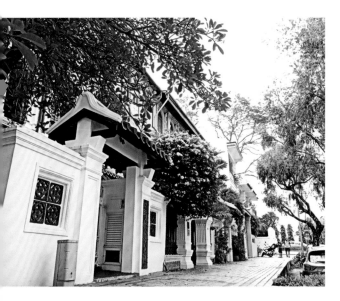
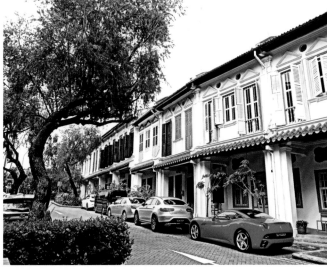

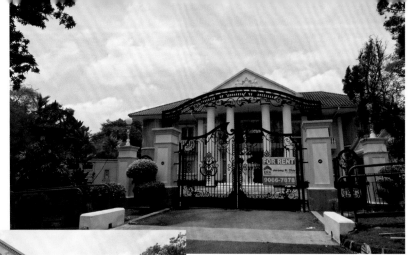

The home belongs to a Singaporean Chinese family, who have moved to an exclusive residential enclave by the sea (a piece of gossip offered by their neighbor, a woman in her sixties). The home is still currently on the market for rent, and it will likely be more difficult to find someone wanting to rent, as flashing cameras outside this home are now a daily affair. The market rate for this neighborhood is asking for around SGD $35,000 (USD $25,000) a month to rent, and approximately SGD $30

Goh Peik Lin's house in the movie *Crazy Rich Asians*

to $40 million (USD $20 to 40 million) to buy. The neighbor gossiped that the rent should be lowered since it has been in the market for a while and she has a few of these homes rented out for much less. Judging from her fifteen-year-old Mercedes and down-to-earth appearance without any trace of makeup or jewelry, she's the exact stereotype of a real Crazy Rich Asian in Singapore—filthy rich but does not look or act the part.

THE STAR TREK HOUSE

Do you remember reading about The Star Trek House in *Crazy Rich Asians*? This is the location where the ladies—led by Eleanor Young—in Carol Tai's mansion enjoy an afternoon of bible studies and a good sharing session. If fact, the afternoon affair is about anything but the bible; the ladies exchange gossip and bless each other's stocks, hoping they will appreciate in value.

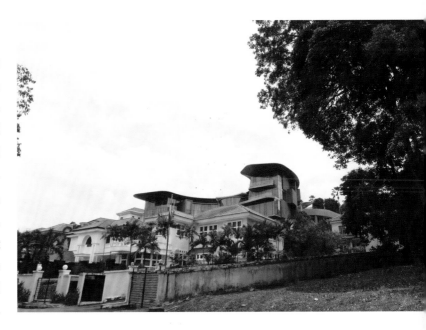

In one of the chapters titled "The Star Trek House," a Christian preacher was claiming almost everything in the house to be satanic. Antique Chinese furniture and porcelain, Ming and Qing dynasty vases and scrolls were all destroyed and thrown away. This is one incident that author Kevin Kwan has mentioned in an interview to be a real event that he personally witnessed.

Here in one of the exclusive neighborhoods in Singapore, there is a giant futuristic home that towers over the entire neighborhood. If a Star Trek–looking home exists in Singapore, this has got to be it.

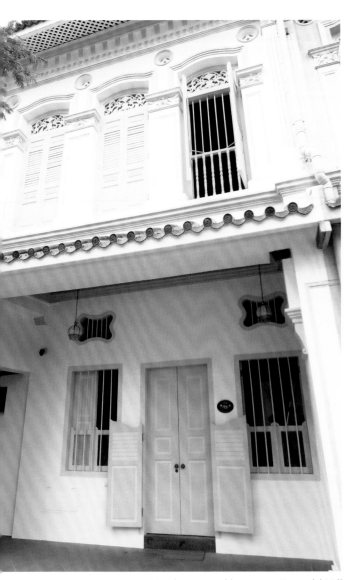

Newly restored home on Emerald Hill

TRADITIONAL PERANAKAN HOUSE ON EMERALD HILL

Right smack in the middle of bustling Orchard Road, our famous shopping district, which is sometimes called "Rodeo Drive on Steroids," there is a quaint and charming neighborhood called Emerald Hill.

The old and traditional shophouse-style homes stick out beautifully among the modern skyscrapers surrounding it. Here in the middle of the bustling city, once you turn off the corner you will find that time moves a little slower and the whole relaxing atmosphere is a nice welcome contrast to the busy malls. More often than not, you will find curious eyes wandering up the hill to check out the beautiful architecture and discover the old and well-preserved quarter.

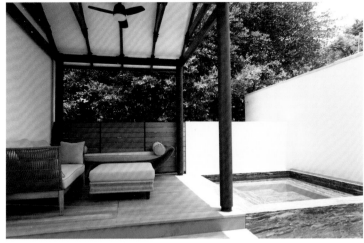
Personal Jacuzzi and patio

It is easy to be fooled into thinking these buildings are small inside as most of them have a very narrow frontage. This is because in the past, the British charged people for the land based on how wide the frontage was, but not on its depth. This is why many of these buildings are narrow in width but go deeper than you'd think and are actually quite spacious. You can sometimes even find a lap pool inside these buildings—they are long enough for that! The common design, however, in all of these shophouses is an air well. One that is extremely important to let sunlight in and to suck out the hot air in tropical Singapore a long time ago when air-conditioning had yet to be invented.

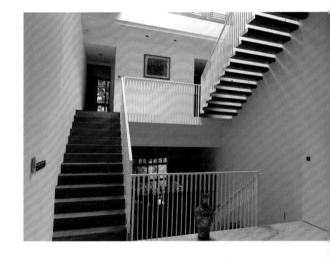

In the second book of the Crazy Rich Asians series, Astrid moved here after leaving her husband and this became Astrid's neighborhood for the rest of the story. Homes here are priced starting from around $5 million to $12 million. If it is good enough for Astrid, it is good enough for anybody!

The home we have featured here is one of the newest families to move into the neighborhood. The family of three lives in the three-story building that has a Jacuzzi pool on the deck of one of the split-levels. This is a great place for the family to have a nice time under the sun.

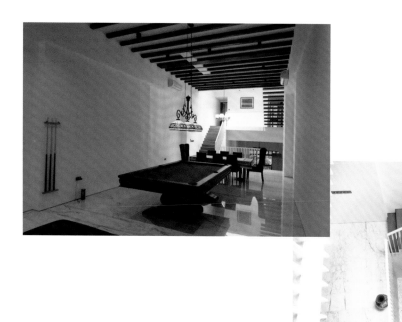

Black and Whites

In the center of the series is Tyersall Park, the beautiful colonial home that belongs to Nicholas Young's grandmother, Shang Su Yi. Said to be located at the back of the Botanic Gardens in Singapore, if there is a real Tyersall Park in Singapore, it will not be too far away from this part of the country.

Historically, there was a beautiful grand palace called Istana Tyersall, which belonged to the late Sultan of Johor, Abu Bakar. It was believed to be the first building in Singapore to be supplied with electricity in 1892. Unfortunately, the palace caught fire several times before it was eventually demolished in the 1930s.

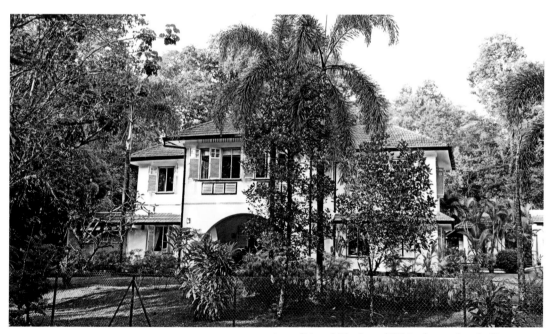

A traditional Black and White bungalow in Singapore

Today, these colonial bungalows that have survived are called Black and Whites because all of them are literally black and white in color. The dark timber beams of the house are painted black, and the walls are painted white. The word "bungalow" came from a Hindi word "banga-la," which means "of, or belonging to, Bengal." Back when India was a British Colony, the British adopted the local way of building homes, adding features like verandas and broad eaves. They later brought this way of building homes to Singapore and Malaysia but made changes to better suit the tropical weather here.

There are about five hundred Black and Whites in Singapore at the moment, and most of them were built between 1900 to the 1930s. The government owns at least half of these homes and all of them have been conserved. It is possible to live in one of these government-owned ones—they are very popular among the expatriate community. Rent for these starts from around $3,000 and can go up to around $25,000 a month.

The privately-owned ones are much more grand in design and are almost never on the market for sale or rent. It is not uncommon to find the privately-owned ones beautifully conserved with new wings added on or even underneath to continue being relevant in the twenty-first century. A glimpse of them can be found in architectural magazines for those that allow their beautiful homes to be admired. *Could there really be a Tyersall Park?*, you might be wondering. It is highly possible, but it will be so secret, the only chance of you getting an invite is to be friends with Rachel Chus dating Nick Youngs, and the period around Chinese New Year will be your best bet.

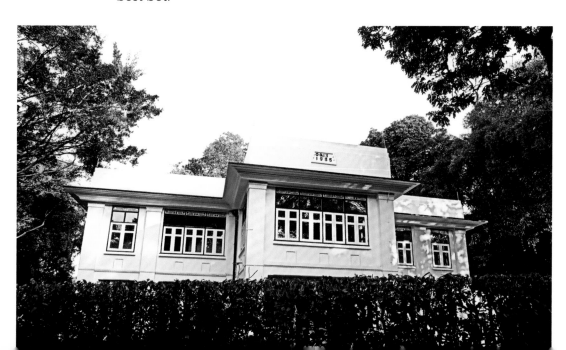

DEMPSEY HILL NEIGHBORHOOD

A formal British Barracks, Dempsey Hill will be familiar to Singaporean men who served in the military in the seventies, as this was the location they had to report for service. Today, this neighborhood has an eclectic mix of retail, lifestyle, and wine-and-dine places, and is one of the hottest locations for finding new restaurants. In the book *Crazy Rich Asians*, this was where Astrid invited Michael to have their first date—and where Michael felt completely out of place. In the third book, Astrid came back here with Nick after an important event and they had a drink at PS. Café .

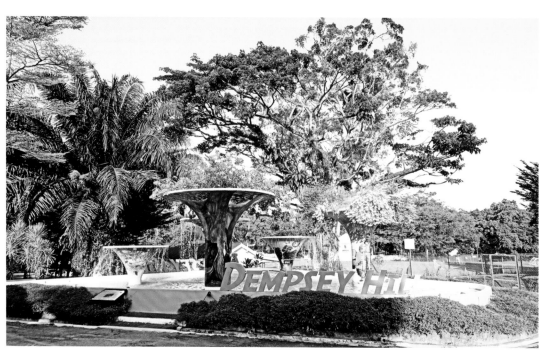

PS. Café at Harding

One of the first places to open on the hill, this is a must-visit especially for a drink or their sinful desserts. The whole café is found in a Black and White house in the forest and the whole vibe of the place is very modern colonial with a lot of beautiful blooms found all around the café, even in the bathroom.

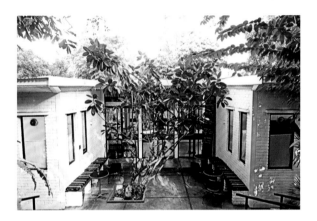

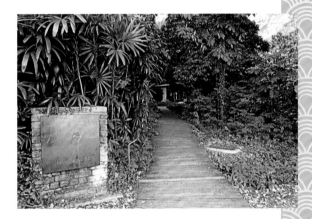

Dover Street Market Singapore

This super cool multi-label boutique from Dover Street in London brings luxury and streetwear fashion to Dempsey Hill. Brought in by Club 21's owner Christina Ong who has the nickname "Queen of Bond Street," this store ups the style of the area by several notches. Long lines of mostly rich kids with spare cash to spend can be seen outside the store whenever a popular new limited-edition sneaker drops.

Open Farm Community

Opened by lifestyle entrepreneur Cynthia Chua of Spa Esprit Group, Open Farm Community offers food that uses ingredients directly from the farm found on site and around Singapore. Local produce is a rarity, as almost everything is imported into Singapore. The space also has a garden, a playground, and a safari tent area offering baked goods and coffee from its bakery.

The White Rabbit

Established in 2008, this restaurant is found right inside a formal chapel. A perfect venue for a date night or a wedding, the tongue-in-cheek signboard outside the restaurant pays homage to the building by reading, "Praise the Lard, Join us for Weekend Brunch."

TIONG BAHRU NEIGHBORHOOD

Built by the former British Government in the 1930s, Tiong Bahru is the first example of public homes in the country. The name of the estate is a fusion word from the Hokkein and Malay language. "Tiong" in Hokkein means "to die" or "in the end" and "Bahru" in Malay means "new." There was a new cemetery nearby in the late 1800s and it was a "new place to die." All of that changed when the estate was built and the government relocated the cemeteries—this became a middle-class neighborhood where many rich men hid their mistresses. Today, the neighborhood has Art Deco–style buildings, and has gone through significant gentrification. It's become a popular place for Caucasian expats to call home and for hipsters to hang out and take photos. British *Vogue* named it as one of the top fifteen coolest neighborhoods in the world.

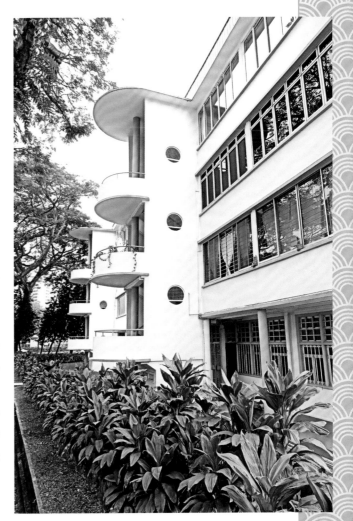

Tiong Bahru Bakery

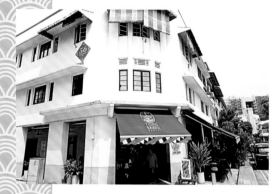

A trip to Tiong Bahru will not be complete without having a sip of the very good coffee and a taste of one of the best croissants in Singapore. All croissants are baked fresh daily and the bakery uses French butter and French flour. This is one of the pioneer hipster places in the neighborhood.

Tiong Bahru Market

Started in 1945, this is the go-to place for food and fresh produce for folks living nearby. You'll find some of the best hawker stalls in the country, and there are constant lines for the popular stalls at lunchtime.

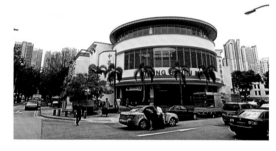

Tiong Bahru Club

This bar found at the heart of the estate is a great place to watch the world go by. Opened in recent years, the bar recreated an old-school vibe to fit into the neighborhood. It's a great place for a drink or two and if you are lucky, you might just spot Prince Charles alighting from his car across the road to go to the market, which he did with his wife in 2018.

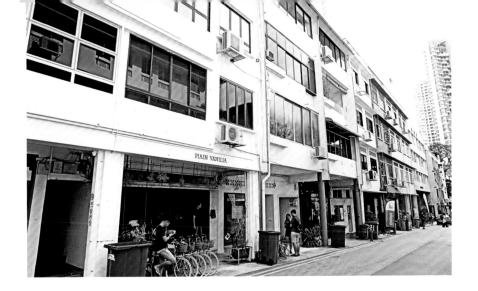

Plain Vanilla

One of the earliest artisanal cupcake shops in the country, this beautiful café has a swing and bicycles at its entrance to create the perfect vibe for a lazy afternoon to munch on a cupcake and watch the world go by.

BooksActually

This is a cute book store with a wide selection and even a book vending machine at its shop front. Take a step back in time and savor the moment, as more and more book stores are sadly disappearing.

Tiong Bahru Qi Tian Gong Temple

The first temple in Singapore dedicated to the Monkey God, the temple opened at the current location in 1938. There are more than ten Monkey God statues at the temple and the oldest one is nearly a hundred years old.

Crazy Rich Fact:
Who Girl That Got $1,000

Good Class Bungalow (GCB) is the most prestigious type of housing in Singapore. Found in prime residential districts in the country, they have strict planning constraints imposed by the government to maintain exclusivity. The minimum land plot size required is 1,400 square meters (or 15,070 sq. ft.) and there is also a maximum building height of two stories. Owners of these homes must follow the strict guidelines, which include not building a home that consumes more than 35 percent of the plot size—this is to maintain sufficient greenery in between plots of land. Reserved exclusively for Singaporeans, foreigners who wish to own landed homes in GCB areas will need to, for starters, become a Singaporean.

There are homes in the market asking for SGD $300 million (USD $220 million) in the Nassim Road area even though there are no takers due to its high price. The most expensive home sold in 2018 was a home sitting on a 42,515 square feet freehold land area. It was sold for SGD $105.3 million (USD $77 million) and this works out to be approximately USD $1,820 per square foot in the exclusive Nassim Road neighborhood. The property was snapped up by the Singaporean chairman of Winson Group, Tony Tung. This is the second property the Tungs have bought on Nassim Road in 2018. A young family member in his twenties also picked up a bungalow down the road and this was at a price of SGD $44 million (USD $32 million). This works out to SGD $2,625 (approximately USD $1,928) per square foot on the land area of 16,765 square feet.

The most sensational sale in recent years, however, was a GCB located along Ridout Road. Not just because the price was a record back in 2015, but also because the drama behind it seems like the storyline right out of a soap opera. Sold for a record SGD $91.68 million (USD $67.3 million), the price for the 73,277 square feet freehold site works out to SGD $1,228 per square foot. The home has been caught up in a ten-year-long dispute among the siblings in the family after their parents died.

This was not the case about half a century ago, though—back then, the Ridout Road house was a happy family home and all the siblings had fond memories of their childhood growing up there. Owned by the late property investor Chow Cho Poon, who owns over twenty properties in Singapore and Australia, the Ridout Road house was home to his family. It was where he and his wife Grace raised four children, three boys and a girl, who grew up playing and studying together, helping each other with school work, and sharing a tight bond. The sprawling estate was huge enough for the siblings to play anything from badminton to a basketball game. Even though they moved away when they grew older, whenever there was a reunion like Chinese New Year, they would come together and spend quality family time in a home filled with happy memories.

Unfortunately, everything changed when their parents died. When Chow Cho Poon died in 1997, he left the family home to his wife and his three sons. His daughter? Betty Sheares was left with just $1,000. This was when things started going south and relationships began to sour. Married to heart surgeon Joseph Sheares, Betty Sheares is the daughter-in-law of Singapore's former president Benjamin Sheares. After their mother's death in 2002, Betty sued the brothers in 2004 and accused them of cheating her of her inheritance. The four siblings have at least six suits involving them and their inheritance and they all went to court for it.

In 2010, a total of nine properties including the office building Chow House were sold for USD $128 million. The home, however, was trickier, as not everyone wanted it to be sold. Second son of the family, architect Kwok Chuen, was against the sale of his family home—he had a strong connection since it was bought by his father in the 1950s. It was also his late mother's wish to keep the property within the family. He had the idea of subdividing the property into four plots and the plot with the family home could be retained since he was unable to buy out his siblings' shares. The huge parcel of land is big enough to be divided into four smaller plots of at least 15,070 square feet and is well within the regulations of the government for Good Class Bungalows.

Items in the house were also fought over by the siblings. These heirlooms include 174 pieces of jewelry and two portraits of their parents drawn by renowned late Singaporean artist Liu Kang.

Today, the three brothers reside in Hong Kong, and the sister in Singapore. The brothers readily speak to reporters about the sad situation of their relationship, but none are willing to speak to each other. There is no more sibling love to speak of, and all of them want to move on quickly from the public dispute and avoid further litigation In the end, the home was sold for SGD $91.68 million (USD $67.3 million), which was above the estimated price. I guess the record price turned out to be the best outcome after the long-drawn-out disagreement. The sold price for the Ridout Road house is higher than it has ever been, so hopefully, money heals all wounds and is the best remedy to unhappiness.

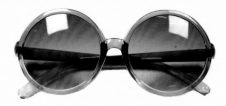

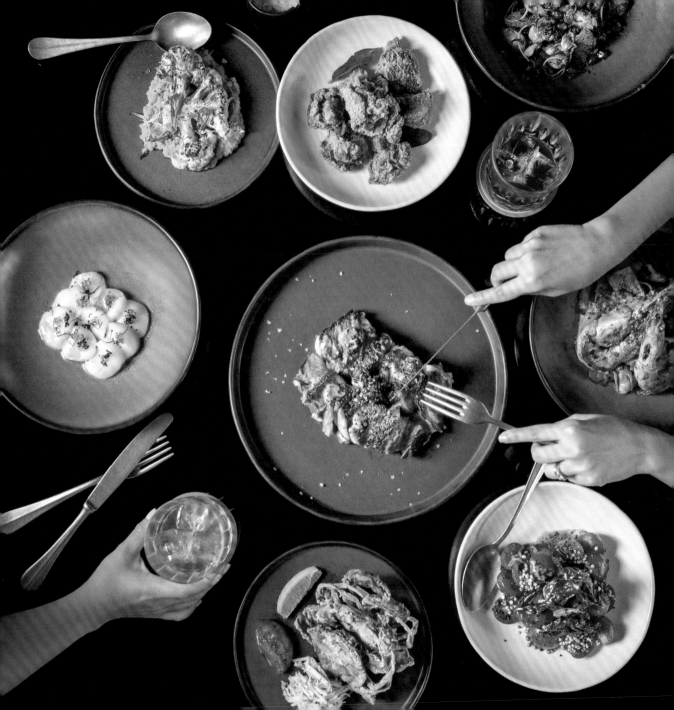

CHAPTER 3:
FOOD

Here in Singapore, we take our food very seriously. From street food found in hawker centers to fine dining in restaurants, everyone has an opinion on what is the best. Even the McDonald's® here are extra hardworking—seeing the same few burgers on the menu will not cut it for Singaporeans and every two to three weeks, they push out a whole set of seasonal offerings.

In this chapter, I'll tell you about one of the newest restaurants found on Dempsey Hill, helmed by famous local chef Ming Tan, as well as some popular local snacks and how to make them, and a few of my favorite places to eat in Singapore.

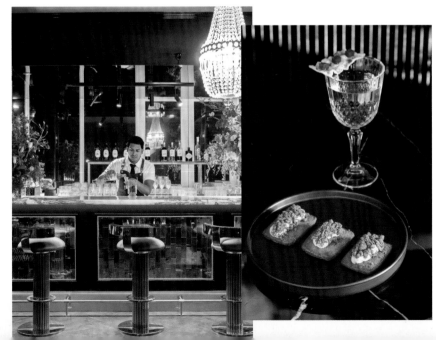

Chicken in a biscuit, spiced cream cheese, chicken skin

Self-Taught Chef Ming Tan

Self-taught chef Ming Tan burst into the Singapore food scene in 2012 when he started out as the head chef of Lolla, a restaurant that, under his direction, was named Top 10 Hottest Restaurants in the World by *Zagat* in 2013. The sea urchin pudding that he created was named the best dish of 2012 by the local papers. The *New York Times* also praise Chef Tan for his spot-on execution as head chef. After his stint at Lolla, Chef Tan together with a few friends opened Park Bench Deli, a hugely popular gourmet sandwich shop that earned him many fans.

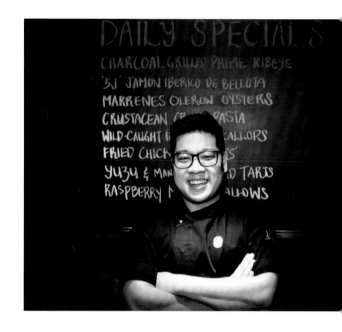

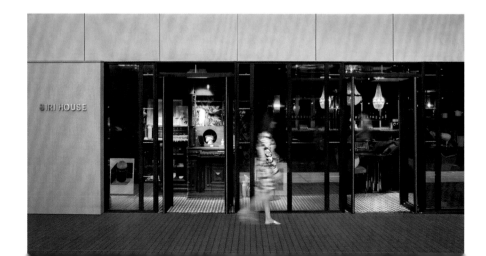

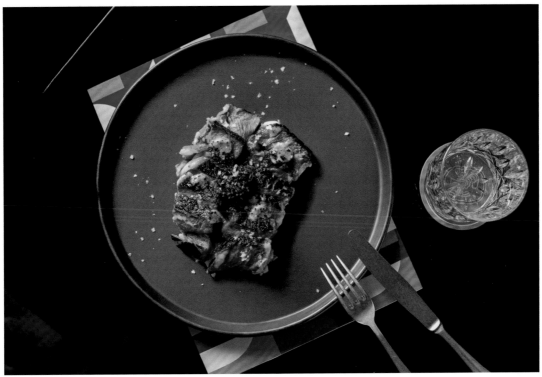

Prime rib with shio kombu butter and salsa verde

His latest project, as head chef of Jam at Siri House, sees him coming together to form a partnership with luxury property developer Sansiri and also Jeremy Cheok, previously from New Ubin Seafood. Chef Tan is bringing to the local food scene something from his heart, not necessarily having a need to be classified as local cuisine, Asian or western. It is an elevated home dining experience that he cooks what he loves, using ingredients and flavors from all genres. It is food for the soul. The possibilities of the food scene in Singapore are endless and Chef Tan is definitely one of the brightest sparks to look out for.

1) What is the concept and direction of Jam at Siri House?

Jam at Siri House aims to create an elevated home dining and drinking experience for our guests. We want to capture that essence of generosity and hospitality guests personally experience at home so everything we do reflects this. Service is warm, friendly, and welcoming, with complimentary surprises from our kitchen at any given moment. We hope to make guests feel like they have been dining with us for years (even if it's their first time here). Sharing plates encourage everyone to tuck in and enjoy a little taste of everything. We've injected fun and playfulness to our menu, taking recognizable favorites and giving them a twist with our own elevated take. Deliciousness is paramount but our plates also celebrate simplicity with a few key elements that highlight the freshness and quality of the produce we carefully source.

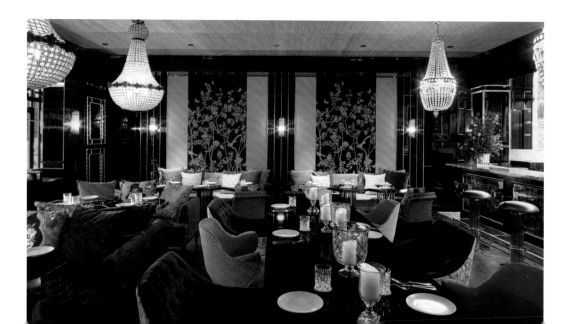

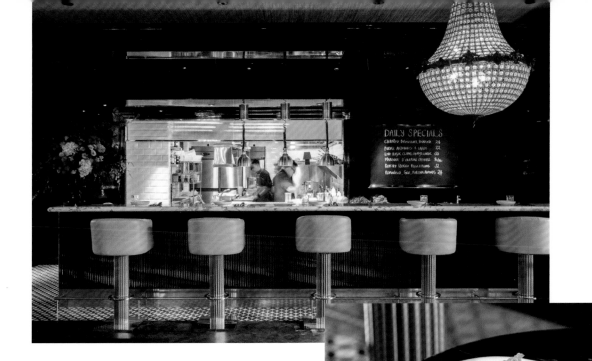

2) What are the inspirations behind the beautiful décor in the restaurant?

Interiors reflect a lovely home. Mid-century antiques juxtapose plush lounge chairs and different fabrics from colorful handwoven silks to Deco jacquard motifs and Chinoiseries fill the room. The space is luxurious, yet comfortable and welcoming at the same time.

3) Who are your target clients?

Our food reflects this idea of accessible luxury which resonates with the modern, well traveled professional cosmopolite.

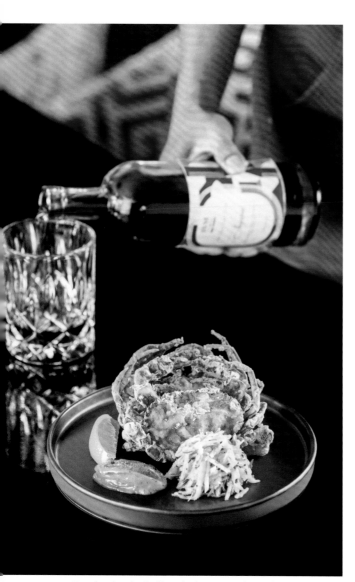

4) What is your favorite local food and where can it be found?
Sin Kee Famous Chicken Rice at Holland Drive! I'm a chicken rice nut.

5) What are the challenges to make it in our local food scene?
Singapore is a great place—but high costs of living mean high staff salaries and rent. We also have a vibrant dining scene that is very competitive, and consumers tend to move quickly between places to dine at because they have such a diverse selection of restaurants to visit. It is not all doom and gloom though, we also have a growing pool of talented local chefs that believe in careers in the food and beverage industry.

Smoked soft shell crab, burnt garlic aioli, jicama slaw

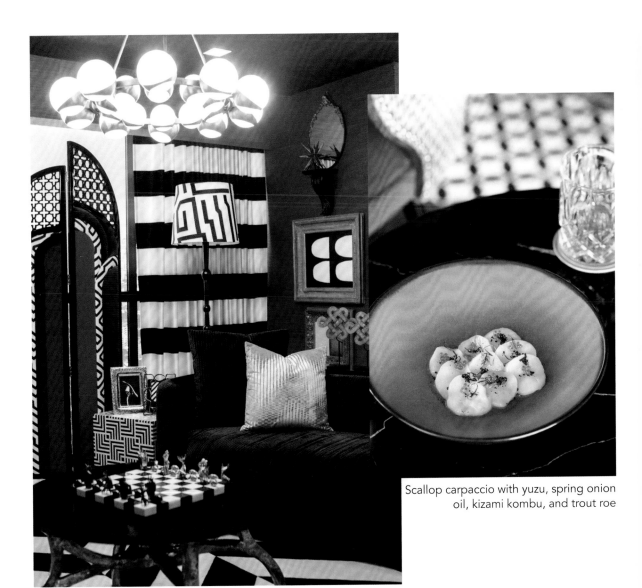

Scallop carpaccio with yuzu, spring onion oil, kizami kombu, and trout roe

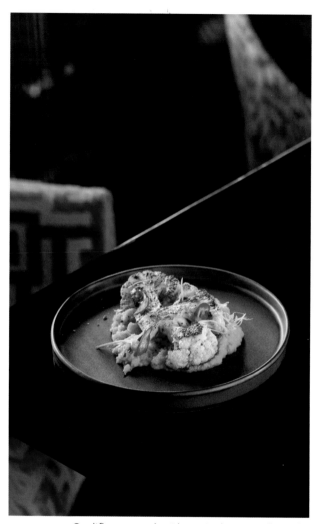

6) What would your last meal be?
Century egg porridge, Hong Kong style roasted meats, and chicken rice. Dessert is an apple pie from McDonald's!

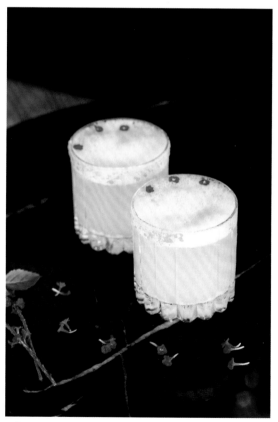

Cauliflower steak with curried carrot, almonds, and sherry vinaigrette

Signature Maize Runner cocktail: roasted coconut whisky, bourbon, peanut froth, corn salt

7) What's your biggest pet peeve as a chef?

My biggest pet peeve has to be famous influencers and celebrities who order a ton of food and drink, complain about it not coming fast enough, then taking six thousand selfies and leaving everything untouched. I die a little each time I see food just sitting, sadly, whilst someone figures out what kind of filter is gonna get them more likes.

8) Are there a lot of Crazy Rich Asians patronizing your restaurant?

Yes. Working in open kitchens means we hear everyone's conversations, and see husbands and wives come in separately with other people, and spend vastly different amounts! We've seen people spend tens of thousands on champagne when they feel in the moment, or when they are trying to impress people.

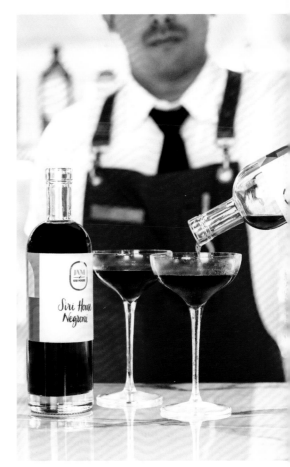

Siri House Negroni

POPULAR SINGAPOREAN SNACKS & RECIPES

Chwee Kueh

As the famous saying goes, don't judge a book by its cover. Be open-minded when trying this famous local snack. A great appetizer or meal on its own, Chwee Kueh is also a popular breakfast item found in many hawker centers in Singapore. For most first-time Chwee Kueh eaters unwrapping the waxed paper they are usually served in, their expressions say, *oh my god, do I really have to try this?* However, one small bite into this famous Teochew cuisine and you will see their faces light up, pleasantly surprised with the delicious taste!

Chwee Kuehs are steamed rice flour cakes topped with preserved radish and also chili sauce on the side. They are simple and hearty, packing a great flavor, and are often the star of a meal at a hawker center.

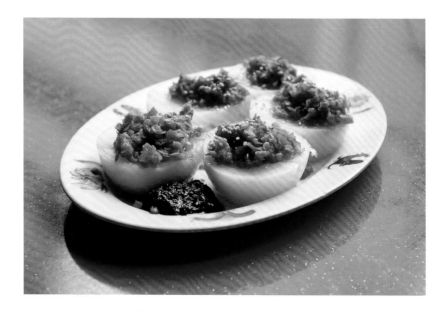

Rice flour cake:

1¼ cups rice flour
2 tablespoons tapioca flour
2 tablespoons corn flour
1 tablespoon salt
1 cup room temperature water
2¼ cups water
   (hot but not boiling)
2 tablespoons vegetable oil

Preserved radish:

1–2 cups preserved radish
2 tablespoons cooking oil
2 shallots, finely chopped
4 cloves garlic, finely chopped
1 tablespoon dark soy sauce
3 tablespoons light soy sauce
4 tablespoons sugar
2 tablespoons toasted white
   sesame seeds
1 tablespoon pepper

Best to pair with sambal chili

Rice flour cake:
1) In a large bowl, mix together the rice flour, tapioca flour, corn flour, and salt.
2) Add the room temperature water to the mix and stir continuously.
3) Add in the 2¼ cups of hot water. This is an important step to stabilize the flour and prevent it from being cooked, but at the same time prevent the water from separating from the flour.
4) Prepare your steamer by bringing a pot of water to a boil. Brush about 20 metal bowls for the rice flour cake with oil. Alternatively, mini muffin tins would work too.
5) Place these empty metal bowls inside the steamer and let steam for 1–2 minutes.
6) Give the batter a stir before dividing into the metal bowls until about ¾ full. Put on the lid for the steamer and steam the cakes on high for 5 minutes.
7) Leave them to cool before scooping the rice cakes out.

continued

Preserved radish:
1) Soak the radish in water for 2 minutes. Drain them, squeezing out as much water as possible. Chop the radish up finely.
2) In a pan, heat 2 tablespoons of cooking oil.
3) Stir-fry the shallots for approximately 2 minutes until they turn soft. Add in the garlic and cook for about 30 seconds. Add the chopped up preserved radish.
4) Add in the dark soy sauce, light soy sauce, sugar, toasted white sesame seeds, and pepper. Stir and combine the mixture until they are dry and fragrant.

Assembly:
1) Scoop the rice flour cakes out of their bowls.
2) Put the preserved radish toppings on top of the rice flour cakes. They will also be perfect with some sambal chili on the side.

Where to get the best Chwee Kueh:

Jian Bo Tiong Bahru Shui Kueh

Started on a push cart at Tiong Bahru Market in 1958, this is arguably one of the best Chwee Kuehs in Singapore and has expanded to become a franchise that has over fifteen stores in the country.

Kaya Toast (Coconut Jam Toast)

A classic Singapore breakfast consists of two pieces of bread slapped with kaya and butter, soft-boiled eggs, and a strong cup of local coffee. The origins of this are a little vague but many believe that during Singapore's rule as a British Colony, the local Chinese saw what the British were eating for breakfast (toast, eggs, and coffee) and decided to create their own version to better suit the Asian palate. To replace strawberry jam, which was most probably too expensive during those times, the locals used a coconut jam infused with the pandan flavor. Pandan juice extracted from the pandan leaves give kaya the green color and also the distinct taste and fragrance.

To give the eggs an Asian twist, soy sauce was added to the soft-boiled eggs instead of salt. Instead of using top-grade coffee beans for espresso, the locals used the cheaper beans and roast them with sugar, oil, and butter. The coffee is usually served with sugar or condensed milk.

Kaya (coconut jam):

8 eggs
1½ cups canned coconut cream
   (I use Kara brand)
½ cup palm sugar

½ cup white sugar
2 tablespoons freshly squeezed
   pandan juice

continued

1) Separate the egg yolks from the whites. It is important to do this carefully to ensure that there are as little egg whites left as possible, so as to avoid lumps in the jam. Using a sieve will help here.
2) Beat the egg yolks with a fork or a whisk until they are smooth.
3) Heat a pan to medium heat and pour in coconut cream, palm sugar, white sugar, and the freshly squeezed pandan juice. Cook the mixture over medium heat and avoid boiling. Stir mixture until the sugar has completely melted.
4) Beat the egg yolks again before adding them into the pan.
5) Stir the mixture over medium heat but do not boil. Stir until it thickens, for at least 20 to 30 minutes.
6) Leave it to cool and the mixture will continue to thicken to become jam-like.
7) The jam is now ready to be bottled up. When placed in the fridge, the jam will be good for at least 2 months.

Kaya Toast:
1) Toast your bread.
2) Spread the kaya jam on freshly toasted bread.
3) Add a thick slice of butter. Some serve the toast with the butter melted and some serve them with the butter still slightly chilled.

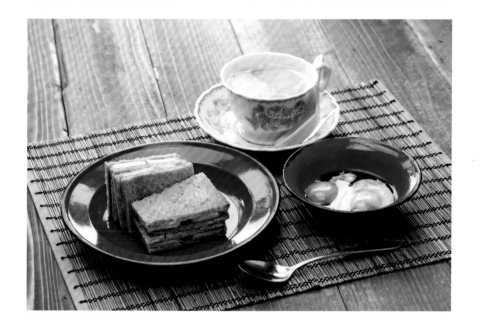

Where to get the best Kaya Toast:

Killiney Kopitiam

Founded in 1919 and nearly a hundred years old, Killiney Kopitiam (Kopitiam means coffee shop, a fusion word created from "kopi" which means "coffee" in Malay and "tiam" which means "shop" in Hokkein) is believed to be the oldest coffeeshop in Singapore today. Renamed in 1993 from "Qiong Xin He," it was the name that everyone calls the place anyway as it is located along Killiney Road. Take a step back in time at this old-school joint and savor the very same style of toast eaten a hundred years ago.

Pineapple Tarts

The pineapple is an auspicious fruit in Chinese culture and is often seen and eaten in various forms during Chinese New Year. The most popular of them all is the pineapple tart, a bite-sized pastry with pineapple jam sometimes found inside the pastries, or on top.

The reason why the pineapple is so popular among the Chinese can be attributed to its golden-yellow color. There's a saying that goes, "everyone loves money, but the Chinese are not ashamed to admit it." For example, the whole Chinese New Year festival has a main theme of money! Instead of getting presents, kids receive money during Chinese New Year. Instead of playing games and sipping hot chocolate, every Chinese family is a gambling den during Chinese New Year. Since the fruit is golden yellow in color and looks auspicious, it is nicknamed "money arriving" by the Hokkeins. In fact, the pineapple fruit is often thrown into a brand-new home or office by the Singaporean Chinese community to bring good luck. It is without a doubt that tarts made with delicious pineapple jam are very popular during festive seasons and throughout the year.

Tart ingredients:

1½ cups pineapple jam
1⅓ cups all-purpose flour
¼ cup milk powder
¼ cup Parmesan or Gouda cheese (shredded)
½ cup butter, room temperature
¼ cup sugar
2 egg yolks

Egg wash:

1 egg yolk, beaten
½ tablespoon honey
½ tablespoon water
½ tablespoon cooking oil

One day prior to baking:

1) Roll pineapple jam into small balls. Combine all egg wash ingredients and brush over the jam balls. Cover and chill in the fridge.
2) In a mixing bowl, combine flour, milk powder, and cheese. Set aside.

Preparing the tarts:

1) Add the softened butter and sugar in the bowl of the mixer and mix until just combined.
2) Add the egg yolks one at a time, creaming together between each addition until just mixed. Switch off the mixer.
3) Add in the flour mixture slowly, mixing with a rubber spatula. (If the dough is dry and does not seem to come together, use clean hands to mix the dough until it forms a ball.)
4) Wrap up the dough and put it in the fridge for 30 minutes.
5) Line a baking sheet with parchment paper.

continued

6) Depending on how many pineapple jam balls you have, divide the dough into the same quantity as the pineapple balls. This recipe should create roughly 35 pineapple tarts. Keep in mind that the dough will expand when baked so try not to make them too big.

7) Use your palm to flatten each of the dough balls and put in the pineapple jam in the middle.

8) Wrap the dough around the pineapple jam—you can get creative how you want them to be shaped. It is popular for the pineapple jam to be in the dough but another popular version is for the pineapple ball to be exposed right on top of the dough.

Baking the tarts:

1) Place the shaped tarts at least 2 inches apart from each other. Put them in the fridge and let them sit for approximately 15 minutes. This step will help with maintaining the shape of the tart.

2) While the tarts are being chilled in the fridge, preheat the oven to 300°F.

3) Place the pineapple tarts on a rack toward the bottom of the oven.

4) Bake them for 20 minutes. They will have a soft and pale appearance.

5) Take them out of the oven and brush more egg wash all over the tarts.

6) Put them back into the oven and continue baking them for another 15 minutes. They should turn golden brown by now.

7) Take them out of the oven and let them sit on the baking sheet for about a minute before transferring them onto the cooling rack to let them cool down further. When they are cooled down completely, they can be stored in air-tight containers and they are good for a month. Put them in the fridge to last longer.

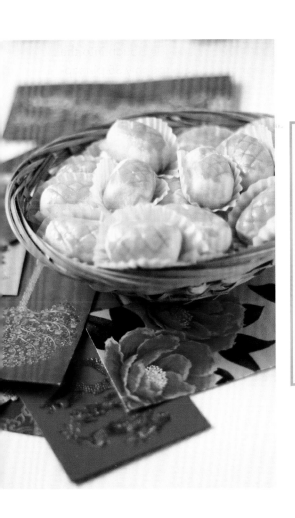

Where to get the best Pineapple Tarts:
Kele Singapore

Opened in 1983, Kele has been in the pineapple tart business for more than thirty years and is frequently voted as "The Best Pineapple Tarts in Singapore." They sell out of pineapple tarts every Chinese New Year, which is the most popular time to eat them.

Ang Ku Kueh (Red Tortoise Cake)

This Red Tortoise Cake, called Ang Ku Kueh in Hokkein, is a hugely popular snack/dessert among Chinese people and is often eaten at celebrations like birthdays or Chinese New Year. This popular Chinese pastry is usually round or oval-shaped. The outer layer is soft and sticky, made with glutinous rice flour, and is usually red in color. Different colors correspond to different sweet fillings in the center. The pastry is molded to look like a tortoise shell, thus the name Red Tortoise Cake. It sits on a square piece of banana leaf and is so popular in Singapore that there is a cartoon character called Ang Ku Kueh Girl. As tortoises have a long life and represent longevity, eating these cakes represents good luck, fortune, and having a long life.

The filling found in traditional Ang Ku Kuehs is usually mung bean or ground peanuts and sugar. However, over the years, bakeries have become creative and it is common today to find fillings like corn, yam, red bean, or pumpkin in modern re-interpretations of this traditional pastry.

Besides being eaten, there is also a Chinese tradition for babies to step on a larger than usual Ang Ku Kueh on their first birthdays. They will have to use their feet to flatten the pastry before wearing a pair of new shoes. This symbolizes them stepping over bad luck and that their future will be a smooth sailing one. This is, however, a fast disappearing traditional rite of passage for babies.

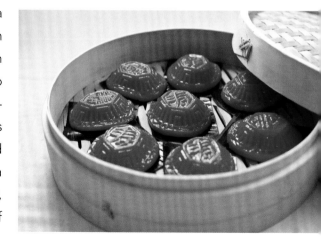

Dough:

5 cups glutinous rice flour
4 tablespoons sugar
½ tablespoon salt
2 cups hot water
¾ cup cooking oil
8–9 drops red food coloring

Filling:

2 cups mung beans
1¼ cups sugar
½ cup cooking oil
2 tablespoons all-purpose flour

Other:

Banana leaves cut into 3x3-inch squares
cooking oil for brushing
Ang Ku Kueh mold

For the dough:

1) Give the glutinous rice flour a good mix together with sugar and salt.
2) Make a hole in the center of the mixture and pour in the hot boiling water.
3) Add in the oil and food coloring. Use a rubber spatula to stir the mixture until it forms a crumbly dough.
4) When the dough mixture has cooled down, knead the dough using your hands into a pliable, shiny, and soft dough.
5) Cover and let the mixture sit for 10 minutes.

continued

For the filling:

1) Soak the beans in water overnight if possible, or at the very least for 1 to 2 hours.
2) Drain the murky soaking water and rinse the mung beans several times until the water is clear.
3) Steam the beans for about 45 to 50 minutes.
4) Add the steamed beans into a blender and blend them until you get a smooth paste.
5) Pour the blended bean paste into a saucepan over medium-low heat. Add sugar. Cook and let the sugar melt into the paste.
6) Add oil to the mixture and stir.
7) Add flour mixture and continue stirring and let it cook until it forms a mass.
8) Allow the mixture to cool down completely.
9) Take about 2 tablespoons of the mung bean filling and roll them into a ball.

Forming the Ang Ku Kueh:

1) Use about 2 tablespoons of dough for each Ang Ku Kueh. Flatten each piece of dough using the palm of your hand.
2) Put the round ball filling in the middle of the flattened dough and bring all edges together. Roll them into a smooth ball.
3) Make sure the Ang Ku Kueh mold is dusted with some rice flour to prevent sticking. Roll the dough ball through the flour as well, to coat lightly.
4) Put dough ball into the mold and gently press to adhere to the mold and take its shape. Then knock the mold on the countertop to get the dough out.
5) Place each Ang Ku Kueh on a greased square banana leaf.

Steaming the Ang Ku Kueh:

1) Get the steamer to boil and place each Ang Ku Kueh an inch apart inside the steamer.
2) Bring down the heat and let it steam for 8 to 10 minutes.
3) Open the lid to allow steam to escape before closing lid back.
4) Repeat this two more times, every 2 minutes. This step is important to ensure the imprints on the cake are maintained and to prevent the Ang Ku Kueh from being flattened. If cake is steamed at high heat, the cake will be flattened and the imprints might no longer be visible.
5) After steaming, remove the Ang Ku Kuehs from the steamer onto a plate before brushing some cooking oil on them.
6) Let the cakes sit and allow them to cool down. Ang Ku Kueh can be eaten warm and at room temperature, and will last for 3 days.

Where to get the best Ang Ku Kueh:

Ji Xiang Ang Ku Kueh

Started in the Kitchen of a public HDB flat in 1985, The Ang Ku Kuehs made by the Toh Family became so popular that they set up a shop at Everton Park in 1988. They were also one of the first to introduce unique flavors like corn, coconut, yam, and durian.

Pandan Chiffon Cake

Do you remember reading about a Chocolate Chiffon Cake at Tyersall Park in *Crazy Rich Asians*? Well, the most famous chiffon cake from Singapore is definitely not a chocolate one but the Pandan Chiffon Cake. If you are wondering what-exactly pandan is, it's a unique flavor derived from a plant that is both fragrant and flavorful, and the pandan juice is green in color.

Eaten by many as a dessert, a snack, or even for breakfast, Pandan Chiffon Cakes are also hugely popular among Hong Kong celebrities visiting Singapore. Famous singers like Andy Lau and Sammi Cheng will always bring back some of these cakes when they visit our sunny city-state. These cakes are also available at a shop in the airport called Bengawan Solo, which has arguably one of the best versions. Besides the pandan version, other famous versions include orange and black sesame. For the chocolate version, you will have to dream about visiting Tyersall Park for it or get down to baking it yourself.

Batter:

6 large egg yolks, room
    temperature
½ cup castor sugar
3 tablespoons cooking oil
½ cup coconut milk
2 tablespoons pandan juice
    (if unavailable, use 2 extra
    tablespoons pandan essence)
2 tablespoons vanilla extract
1 tablespoon pandan essence
1 cup sifted cake flour
2 tablespoons baking powder
¼ tablespoon salt

Meringue:

9 egg whites from large eggs
1 tablespoon cream of tartar
½ cup castor sugar

For the batter:

1) In a bowl, whisk together the egg yolks with the castor sugar and cooking oil.
2) Add coconut milk, pandan juice, vanilla, and pandan essence.
3) In another mixing bowl, combine the cake flour, baking powder, and salt.
4) Slowly add the flour mixture to the egg batter while mixing. Make sure that the mix
    is smooth with no visible lumps. If needed, strain the batter to remove any lumps.

For the meringue:

1) Place the egg whites in a clean bowl and beat until frothy.
2) Add cream of tartar and beat until it turns almost white in color.
3) Add the castor sugar a bit at a time and continue beating.

continued

4) Beat the mix until the meringue starts to hold its shape when you bring up the whisk. This should take at least 5 minutes.

5) Add a quarter of the meringue into the thick batter. Gently fold the mixture from side to side, using a rubber spatula and allowing it to mix.

6) Add in another quarter and repeat the mixing steps above until the batter and meringue are well mixed up.

Baking the Pandan Chiffon Cake:

1) Place the oven rack in the third spot from the top and preheat the oven to 330°F.

2) Do not grease the chiffon cake tin as the cake needs to cling to the tin to rise. Pour in your batter.

3) After adding in the batter, smooth over with a rubber spatula. Give the cake tin a few strong taps to remove any air bubbles. Another way is to use a toothpick to remove the air bubbles.

4) Place the cake tin in the oven and allow it to bake for approximately 55 minutes. Don't open the oven door in the first 30 minutes of baking, as it will cause the cake to be deflated. If there are cracks on the top of the cake, it is perfectly fine since that will actually be the bottom of the cake.

5) After removing the cake tin from the oven, invert the tin upside down and allow it to cool completely. This usually takes at least 2 hours. It is important to not attempt removing the cake from the tin while it is still warm.

6) When ready, use a spatula knife to move it through the edge of the cake to help remove it from the tin.

7) Gently push and tap the base of the cake tin to push the cake out. If needed, use the spatula knife once again to aid in the removal of the cake from the cake tin. The cake will be good for 3 days.

Where to get the best Pandan Chiffon Cake:

Bengawan Solo

Founded in 1979 in the home kitchen of a public HDB flat, Bengawan Solo's Pandan Chiffon Cake is one of the best in the country and is found at every airport terminal in Singapore as they make great gifts. There are now more than forty locations island wide and the familiar flavors of the cake can easily be found in almost every neighborhood.

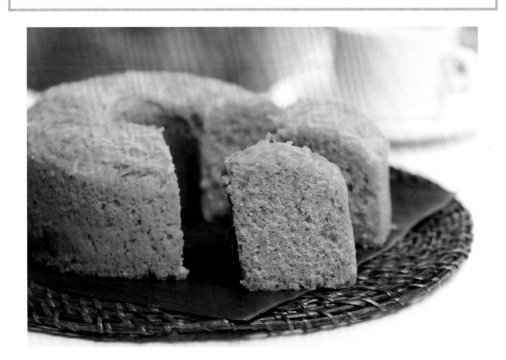

Must-Try Singaporean Specialties

Wee Nam Kee Hainanese Chicken Rice Restaurant

This was mentioned in *China Rich Girlfriend* as the place Eleanor would go because parking is $2.20 after 6:00 p.m. However, this place has been around since 1989 and serves really good chicken rice, much better than the most expensive chicken rice in Singapore at Chatterbox, where every Indonesian Chinese just want to be seen and every Japanese tourist want to say they have eaten there.

MUST-TRY: *White Chicken Rice/noodle set, Dumpling Soup*

National Kitchen by Violet Oon

Rumored to be invited by the government to open at the National Gallery as we needed a restaurant serving local cuisine in our grand old monument. Prime Minister Lee Hsien Loong has dined here several times, inviting people like Australia's Ex-Prime Minister Tony Abbott and a Thai princess. Apparently, our Prime Minister cannot eat too much spicy food, as we were told he ordered a Dry Laksa and was sweating buckets! This place is a must-visit to discover Singapore's unique Peranakan cuisine. Beautiful décor and vibe, unpretentious food sharing creating a casual joyous air in the restaurant—not to be missed if you can secure a table!

MUST-TRY: *Gado Gado, Kuay Pie Tee, Satay, Cod in Creamy Laksa Sauce, Daging Chabek Beef Cheek, Chap Chye, Meatless Meatballs Rendang, Pulot Hitam with Coconut Ice Cream*

Scissors Cut Curry Rice

Perfect place for a late-night supper. In fact, this place made headlines because a local actor came here for takeout after a night of partying at the clubs, and knocked somebody down with his car and drove off. He was given jail time and also got his license revoked. Guess he will not be eating this for the rest of his life. If you are wondering about the name, it's because everything served will be cut up with scissors. Here, you pick the dishes you want and the employee will cut them up before drowning everything with curry and some special sauce. It tastes better than it looks.

MUST-TRY: *Braised Pork Belly, Goh Hiang, Tau Pok, Cabbage, Egg, Luncheon Meat with Tomato Sauce*

Beach Road Prawn Noodle House

This place is packed at lunchtime and the current outlet is found along East Coast Road instead of what its name suggests. Sells a very good version of the prawn noodle and my personal favorite is the dry one instead of the soup version. Try the pigtails if you are adventurous, they taste really good!

MUST-TRY: *Prawn with Pork Ribs and Pigtail Dry Prawn Noodle with Extra Chili, Century Egg*

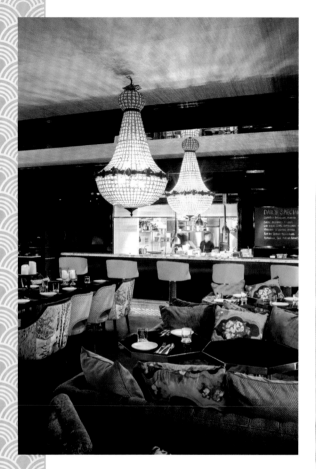

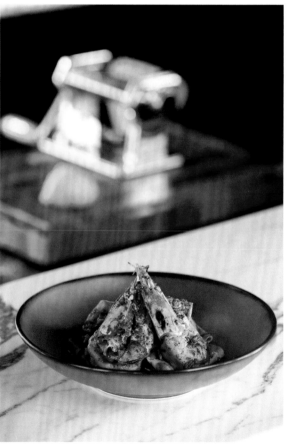

Ban Leong Wah Hoe

Jumbo Seafood is great, but if you want something more local and authentic, "tze char" which means "cook and fry" is a type of restaurant found all around the island at very reasonable prices. They fire up the wok to cook dishes on demand and will sometimes remind people of home-cooked meals. Here at Ban Leong, which was founded in 1986, a lot of local celebrities would patronize this place because it is relatively near the old television broadcasting station. The fuss-free and unpretentious vibe will welcome you even if you are wearing your Sunday's worst. It is located next to the beautiful Pierce Reservoirs with monkeys at the roadside. A walk in the park after your meal can be a great thing to do to burn off some calories and also to say hi to the monkeys.

MUST-TRY: *Sambal Kang Kong, Chili Crab with Golden Fried Buns, Black Pepper Crab, Pork Ribs King, Prawn Paste Fried Chicken, Tofu with Seafood*

Janice Wong Singapore

For the most unexpected chocolate flavors, check out Janice Wong chocolates. They taste as good as they look and they are excellent gifts. Named Asia's Best Pastry Chef more than once by San Pellegrino Asia's 50 Best, Janice Wong also makes edible art by transforming art studios with her installations such as marsh-mallow ceilings and gum drop covered walls. Her restaurant at the National Museum is also decorated with Janice Wong's edible creations. Her restaurants can now be found in Singapore, Tokyo, and Macau, and her stores can be found in Singapore and London.

Crazy Rich Fact: The Car on Display

Imagine buying a brand-new supercar that hits the century sprint in 3.2 seconds but all you can do is admire it and not be able to drive it. . . . That's exactly what a Singaporean businessman is willing to do so that he can be one of the twenty-one in the world to own a Lamborghini Reventon Roadster. He is, however, not the only lucky Singaporean to have his hands on the supercar. Rumor has it, there were three Lamborghini Reventon Roadsters delivered to Singapore, and we might just be the country with the highest density of exotic supercars in the world.

Singapore is the most expensive country in the world to own a car, and there are good reasons behind it. It is a country so small that on the world map, it is merely a tiny red dot, and some are unsure of its location. From the west side of the country to the east side, it is approximately 50 kilometers and a traveling duration of about forty minutes. This is why in a country with 5.6 million people, if everyone owned a vehicle and drove it daily, the whole country would be shut down and unable to move. To avoid the jam situation that many other Southeast Asian cities are facing, the government introduced measures to make sure that unless a person really needs a car and has a lot of spare cash, a car will be a luxury good out of reach to the regular joe. There are heavy taxes slapped on cars upon entry into the country. The taxes include the following: registration fee, road tax, Certificate of Entitlement (COE), tiered Additional Registration Fee (ARF), and customs duty. That is a lot of money bleeding from your wallet just to own a car. The COE, for example, is a certificate one has to purchase to drive a car on the roads for ten years. This means after ten years, a new certificate needs to be purchased and the price of it depending on supply and demand can start from around $20,000 to $100,000.

With only about 600,000 private cars on the roads in Singapore, zipping around town on a regular day is quite easy and breezy. Most cars are clean and new because if you have to pay an arm and a leg for a car, you can probably afford to keep it nice. A 2019 Toyota Prius in Singapore costs SGD $140,000 (USD $105,000). Such a price tag will get you a Mercedes S500 in the United States. Almost everyone buying a new entry-level Japanese or Korean car in Singapore will be able to afford to zip around in a Porsche Macan in other countries.

This is why owning a supercar in Singapore is not just for the rich but for the ultra-rich. All brand-new Ferraris, Lamborghinis, and Rolls-Royces have price tags above $1 million in Singapore. Owning a rare supercar such as the Lamborghini Reventon Roadster sets you back about $2 million. To drive it on the road? A whopping SGD $5 million (USD $3.67 million) after paying taxes. This is why the famous owner of one of these cars puts it on display at the front of his house for the world to see, but will be unable to drive it as the car has not been registered for road use. If you are ever in the exclusive neighborhood of Tanglin, keep your eyes open and you might just be able to spot the rare beast.

Singaporeans are sometimes numb to a regular Ferrari or Lamborghini, as we see nice cars all the time. However, this is also a country which is home to some of the rarest supercars, and some of them will definitely turn heads.

Only forty of the Pagani Zonda S Roadster were made in the world, and one of them managed to make it to our shores. It has a price tag of USD $1.76 million in Singapore after taxes. This is a first Zonda to feature a convertible roof; the one delivered here was yellow in color originally but subsequently painted pink, most likely as a present for a lucky girl's sweet eighteenth birthday.

Another Pagani, the Zonda Cinque, is estimated at USD $2.89 million in Singapore. This is a car that is said to be the most extreme road-legal Zonda ever created in its history. Five were built in the world and the word on the streets is that one of them has been spotted thundering down our roads before.

The most expensive car in Singapore was registered in 2013—a Koenigsegg Agera S estimated at USD $3.89 million. This is once again a very rare one-in-five to ever be built in the world and a proud lucky owner here has the car in his garage.

Can it get crazier? The current title for the most expensive car in Singapore goes to the big bad sibling of the last record holder Koenigsegg Agera S. Around 2016, a Koenigsegg Agera RS estimated at a whopping USD $5 million was purchased and registered in Singapore. This is just one of twenty-five made in the world and will definitely make your heart skip a beat if your bus happens to pull up beside it at the traffic light.

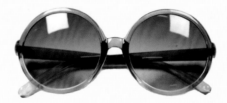

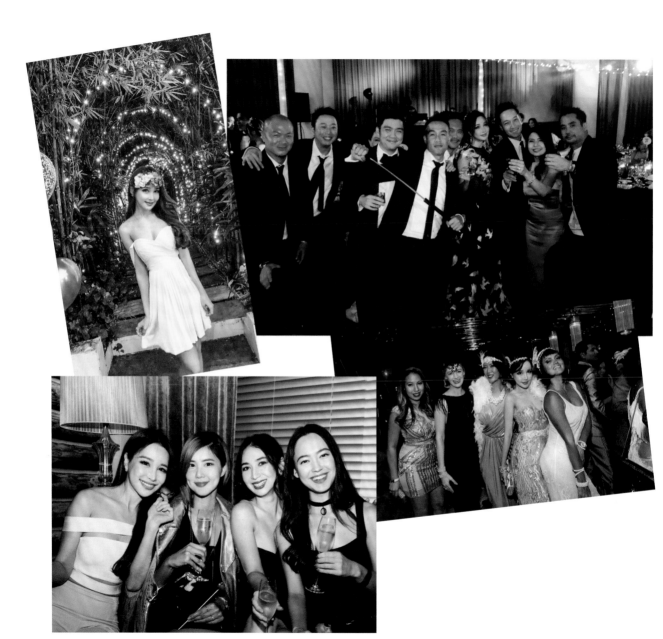

CHAPTER 4:
PARTIES & FASHION

LIFE OF THE PARTY

Dawn Yang first burst into the local scene after her blog became the talk of town. She was one of the pioneer celebrity bloggers before Instagram and Facebook, before there was the hashtag #RKOI (Rich Kids of Instagram). Back then, she went by the moniker "ClapBangKiss" and her blog entries gained attention because of her good looks and her envious lifestyle. Having attended some of the best local schools like Singapore Chinese Girls' School and Raffles Junior College, Dawn went on to further her education in the United States at NYU and could be seen on her blog speeding into the sunsets in her convertible sports car when she was nineteen years old.

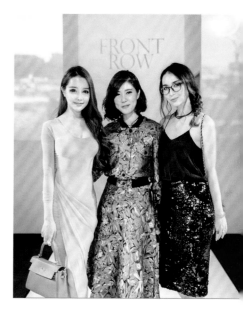

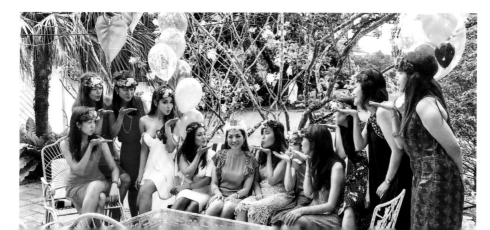

Today, Dawn is the life of the party and super-famous, attending society events and parties and can be found jet setting around the world in her leisure time. She also runs a very successful online fashion store called Lexi Lyla, and she models her creations on her Instagram account @dawnyang.

Here we'll let the photos do the talking and let Dawn take us to the party!

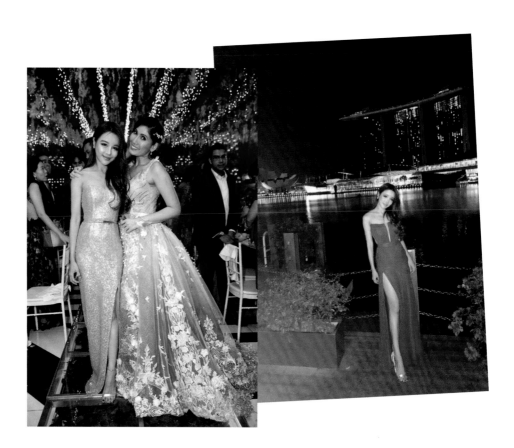

LOCAL FASHION BRANDS

Charles & Keith

Charles and younger brother Keith started working in their parents' humble shoe store in Ang Mo Kio before opening their first shop in 1996. In 2011, LVMH invested 20 percent to help the brand expand globally. Today, there are more than three hundred stores worldwide and the brand has a global footprint across Asia, Europe, Latin America, Africa, and the Middle East.

KNOWN FOR: *Shoes and bags*

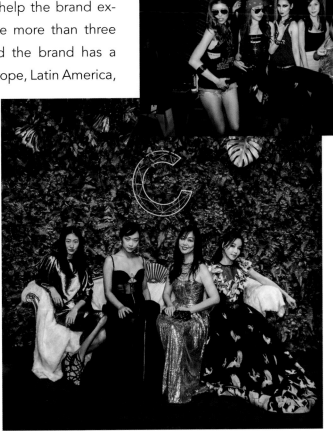

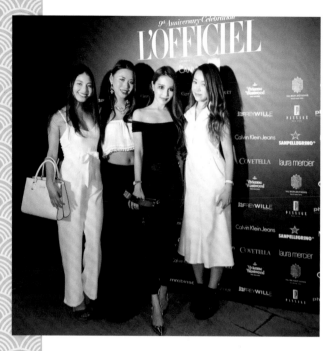

LAICHAN

At Paragon Shopping Centre, you will not find the L'Orient Jewelry mentioned in *Crazy Rich Asians*, but you can certainly find Astrid shopping at LAICHAN for a gown or Cheongsam to wear to a party. Touted as Singapore's Cheongsam Grandmaster, Lai Chan opened Singapore Fashion Week in 2017 and has over thirty years of experience in his craft. The Cheongsam Maestro's creations are hand-stitched with care and attention to details. His designs are modern and current, giving a playful twist to the classic Cheongsam.

KNOWN FOR: *Cheongsams*

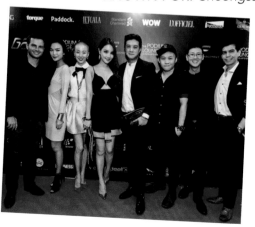

Carrie K.

Started in 2009, the brand was established out of love for meaningful storytelling behind its jewelry. Carrie K. offers affordable luxury with unique and contemporary designs.

KNOWN FOR: *Jewelry*

RISIS

The family-owned brand is known for its 24-karat gold-plated natural orchids with outstanding quality. Started in 1976, they can be found at the Botanic Gardens after your visit to the beautiful Orchid Garden. This is one of the best gifts to take home from Singapore as Orchids represent Singapore and these gold-plated ones are timeless. The brand is owned by the BP de Silva Conglomerate, one of the oldest family businesses in Singapore—it's close to 150 years old and has a stake in Swiss watch brand Audemars Piguet.

KNOWN FOR: *24-karat gold-plated orchid jewelry*

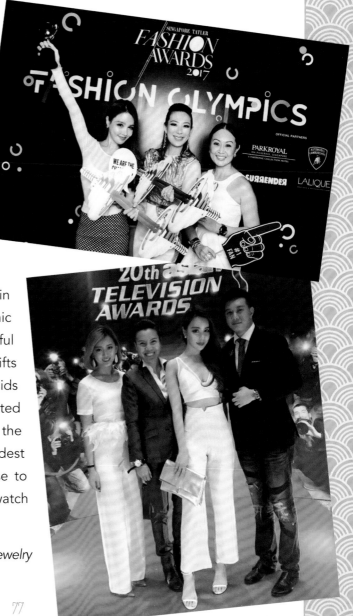

Our Second Nature

Founded by Velda Tan, who was a pioneer in online retail shops in Singapore when she started Love, Bonito, a fast fashion brand that has a huge following. She is also the founder of her other brand Collate the Label, which is now sold exclusively online. Our Second Nature offers effortlessly chic, comfortable women's wear and can be found at Chip Bee Gardens, an old laid-back neighborhood with quaint cafés and charming boutiques.

KNOWN FOR: *Effortlessly chic and comfortable womens wear*

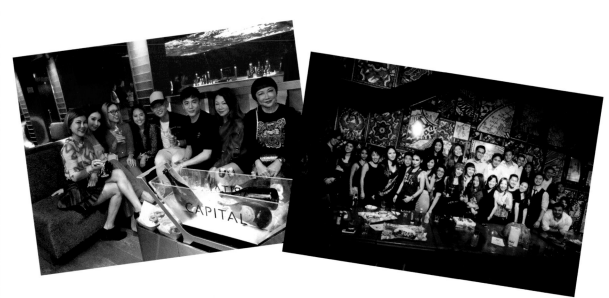

Ethan K

The barely-ten-year-old brand has celebrities like Elizabeth Hurley wanting their hands on an Ethan K bag, priced between $4,000 to $25,000. Found stocked in many exclusive department stores in the world like Harrod's in London, Galeries Lafayette in Paris, Saks Fifth Avenue in Los Angeles, and of course in Singapore, Ethan Koh started attracting attention to his creations when he carried his bags around London while studying there. It is no wonder that the finest eyes are drawn to the quality of his croc-odile bags because he has access to one of the best sources in the world. His father and grandfather started Heng Long Tannery in 1977 and supply crocodile leather to brands like Hermès and Louis Vuitton. The business grew so big that LVMH (Moët Hennessy–Louis Vuitton SE) bought a controlling stake in their company in 2011 for $161 million. The company is among the top five exotic skin tanneries in the world and pro-cesses more than a quarter of a million crocodile and alligator skins every year. If you own a crocodile bag, there is a high chance the skin was dyed and processed in Singapore.

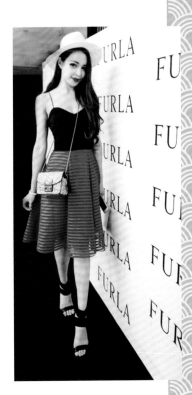

KNOWN FOR: *Bespoke handmade Crocodile-skin bags, each taking seven to eight months to make*

Crazy Rich Fact:
Friend of Ronaldo

Kim Lim, billionaire heiress, philanthropist, fashionista, influencer, and mother to her adorable son, Kyden. A life envied by many; a glimpse into Kim Lim's life on social media is closely followed by 260,000 of her fans and the media cannot get enough of her.

Born with good looks and a platinum spoon, Kim is endearing to her fans because she is down to earth but can also be ultra-glamorous. On some days, Kim can be found makeup-free in shorts and slippers dining at a street-food stall but on another day, she can be seen dressed to the nines in society magazines and rubbing shoulders with celebrities.

The down-to-earth heiress has no airs about her due to her upbringing and her father's constant reminder for her to stay humble. In fact, she was unaware that her father is a billionaire until she was around seventeen years old. How did she find that out? By reading it from the newspapers. Her dad has always wanted her and her brother's childhood to be as normal as possible, despite their wealth.

Kim's father, Peter Lim, is one of the wealthiest men in Singapore. In 2018 he had a net worth of approximately SGD $2.4 billion according to *Forbes Singapore*. A big fan of football, Peter Lim owns Spanish football club Valencia, image rights to Cristiano Ronaldo, and even a hotel right beside Manchester United Stadium. His favorite car? Most probably a McLaren since he has a stake in the automotive brand as well. Peter Lim is also a great inspiration for many who want to make it big, as he has a real-life rags-to-riches story. Son of a fishmonger, Peter Lim worked many jobs before earning the title of the "Remisier King of Singapore." He has worked as a waiter, a cook, and a taxi driver. With his hard-earned money, he also put himself through school and eventually got to where he is today.

Peter Lim's affinity with football has made him friends and business partners with some of the most famous football players in the world. On a regular day in Singapore at a city fringe mall Great World City, spotting David Beckham in a restaurant might cause a person to hyperventilate and faint. It would be a meal to remember for life—but for the Lim family, to have David Beckham as your lunch buddy is a regular thing whenever the world-famous football star sneaks into town.

Kim's pregnancy back in 2017 was kept under wraps until a famous football star visited her and broke the news to the world, with rumors spreading like wildfire about who the baby's father was. For a normal person, having a visitor probably wouldn't cause a media frenzy, but in Kim's case, the visitor was none other than Cristiano Ronaldo. He wore a blue cap and shades, but these were not enough to shield the handsome footballer from being recognized by the public at Thomson Medical Centre, one of the top private hospitals in Singapore owned by none other than Kim's father, of course. Millions of fans would kill for a photo with Cristiano Ronaldo, but on that day, Ronaldo only wanted a photo with Kim, but got rejected because of her insecurities about her pregnancy weight gain.

Having a private jet at the tip of your fingers and being able to fly to anywhere in the world is just one of those things that makes Kim Lim a real-life Crazy Rich Asian. She does not, however, just use that privilege for herself. The heiress was also a heroine to Korean superstar Seungri from pop boyband BigBang when he was stuck in Bali. There was a volcano eruption and Bali airport was closed with all flights grounded. Upon finding that out, Kim, being the sweetest friend and a hero for her friend in need, sent her plane to rescue the K-pop star. It would be hard to imagine with all the privilege in the world that Kim takes the bus and rides the subway sometimes in Singapore. The heiress has taken the MRT (Mass Rapid Transit) train and also the bus with friends when she was younger. She can even provide the bus number without hesitation and is a true-blue humble princess.

With all the public scrutiny, her life was almost in danger in 2014 when she and her brother were scoped out by kidnappers. It ended up being a close shave as the kidnappers decided to choose an easier target, an elderly mother of a supermarket chain's boss. This is why Kim has security following her around and that she goes to great lengths to keep her adorable son Kyden's identity private and away from social media.

The next big event for Kim will most likely be her wedding, which has been postponed twice. The first time was in March 2018 with invitations already sent out, but it got derailed when she got pregnant. She had planned to hold the wedding of the year at the end of 2018 but it got canceled once again because she hadn't reached her ideal weight. Like every girl that dreams of having the perfect wedding and being the most beautiful bride on their wedding day, Kim is no different and will work toward realizing that dream. The only difference? She can postpone it again and the world will wait because, in Kim's world, the possibilities are endless.

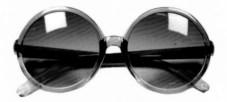

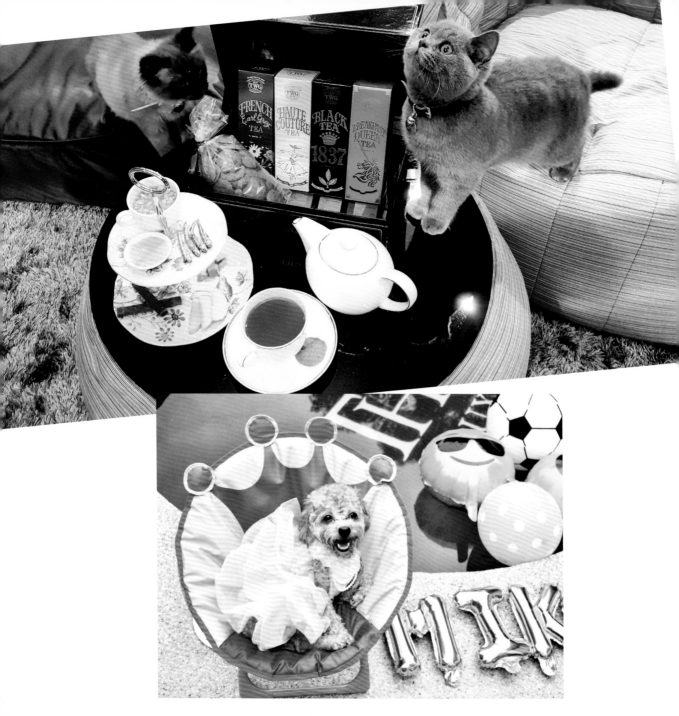

CHAPTER 5:
PETS

The Wagington Luxury Pet Hotels & Resorts

"If your dogs are into watching television, we do have pets' movie entertainment in our double bed Royal Suite," Mya said cheerily while giving us a tour.

Welcome to the Wagington, a luxury pet hotel located in one of the most prestigious neighborhoods in Singapore, Dempsey Hill. The 1920s black and white two-story colonial bungalow has twenty-seven suites and is a five-star premium luxury experience. Here at the hotel, happy pet owners can leave their best friends in the care of pet angels like Mya for a few hours or even for weeks if they are going on a holiday. The pets will be so pampered that when you return, they might not even want to leave with you to go back home.

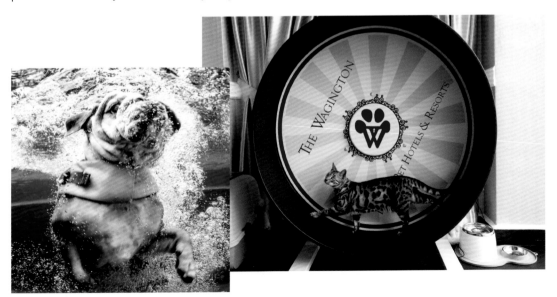

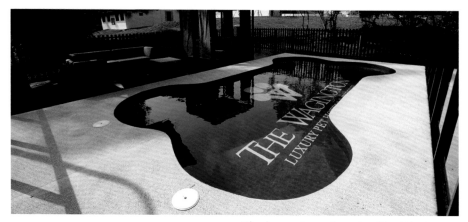

The bone-shaped pool at The Wagington

Estelle Tayler, owner of the hotel says they cater to an exclusive market who do not mind splashing top dollars on their pampered furballs. She invested $700,000 in the business and has her own dog, Bobo, an English bulldog, as the face and mascot of the Wagington.

Tayler explained, "We have a clean beautiful home, a comfortable bed when we are away—your best friend should be left in a place that's just like home. If we deserve the best in life, shouldn't your most loyal companion deserve it equally?"

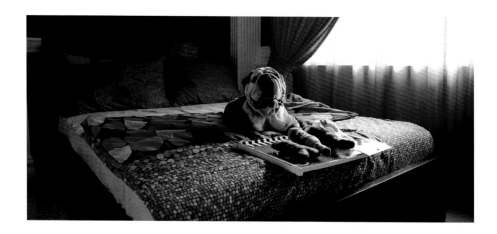

Facilities include a bone-shaped pool, where champagne parties (for the humans) can be held and the dogs can frolic in the water and get some sun. After the party, if showering and drying your fur kids is too much work, leave it to the good hands of the pet stylists at the Wagington's W Salon & Spa. For an indulgent experience, the signature treatment at the spa uses Dead Sea mud from Jordan to give your pooches a good massage, leaving them with beautiful skin and rejuvenating their mind and spirit after their workout in the pool. There are four types of mud masks to choose from to suit all skin types and other treatments include aromatherapy facial and head massage and "Pawdicure."

The Wagington also has a fitness specialist to help get your pets in shape while enjoying an array of fun activities designed just for them. For example, there is treadmill training and bicycle riding sessions to help your pampered pets squeeze into their party dress.

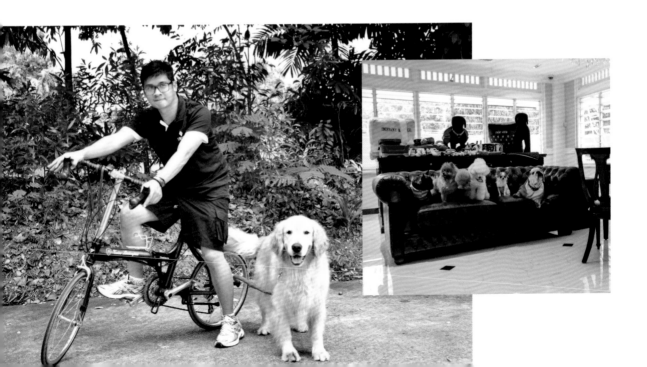

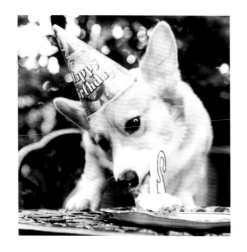

Birthdays, wedding solemnization, any celebrations are all possible at the Wagington! The bone pool is perfect for a pool party as the fur kids can have fun in the pool and under the sun while the proud parents sip champagne and enjoy canapes. For the kitty lovers, having English afternoon tea can be the *purrfect* way to spend the afternoon with your feline friends.

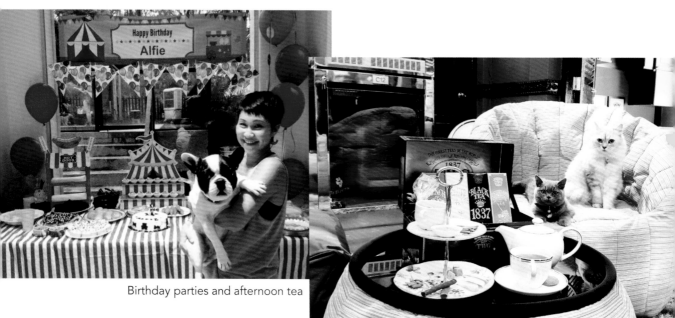

Birthday parties and afternoon tea

From day care to the Royal Suite, there is something for everybody at the Wagington. There are four types of suites for the pooches and five different types for the felines. In-room dining is also available in all suites. The Royal Suite is the most well-appointed accommodations at the hotel offering only the finest for your pampered best fur kids. The elegant proportions of the suite, the stately furnishings and the beautiful artwork of Royal Blue classical interior come together to make The Royal Suite literally fit for a king. The suite offers pet guests 96 square feet of comfortable living space, a privacy glass door, and a queen-sized bed. The suite also comes adorned with a beautiful chandelier that allows for individual mood lighting control to provide your fur kids with the environment that best suit them and also the ultimate relaxation at the end of the day. A 32-inch LED TV can also be found in the suite for guests to indulge in a movie or two. During their stay, they will also be able to enjoy an array of gourmet selections from the in-room dining menu.

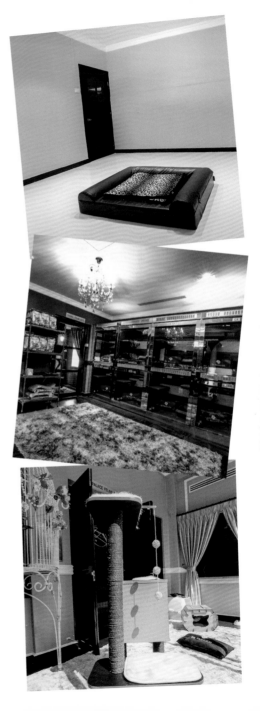

The lovely purrfect Palace Feline Suite offers our feline guests the wonderful view of Dempsey Hill right at the main entrance of the Wagington. This stylish suite at a hundred square feet features an elegant classic decor. There is a huge beautiful bird cage with gorgeous flowers to give the feline guests of this room a feeling of being in an enchanted garden. The spacious suite allow its occupants plenty of room to relax and stretch out, a purrfect getaway for larger families or long stay guests.

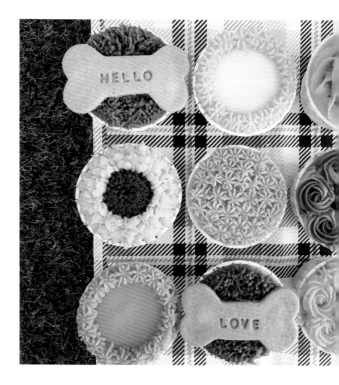

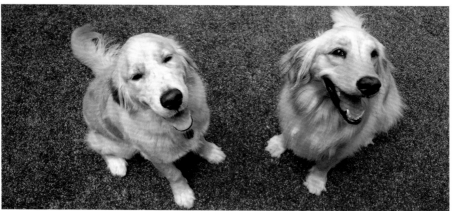

GOURMET PET FOOD—FEED MY PAWS

Worried that her fur kids were not getting the best nutrition from the store-bought pet food, and unsure about the unhealthy ingredients and preservatives found in them, Crystle Tan, founder of Feed My Paws, decided to start making daily meals and treats for her dogs herself. As a fabulous chef and a foodie, she experimented with different ingredients and created an exciting cat and dog-friendly menu of human-quality ingredients.

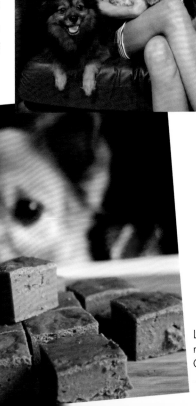

Liver fudge dog treat recipe created by Crystle Tan

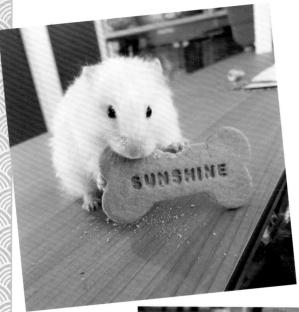

From exotic local delights such as durian tarts, mooncakes, and unicorn cupcakes, to classics such as casseroles and meatloaf, she's constantly looking for new items to add to the menu so that dogs and cats get to enjoy what their owners do too!

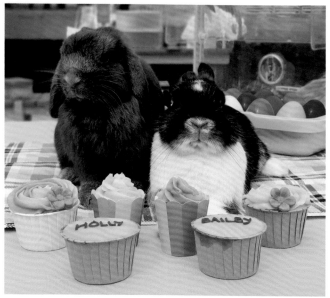

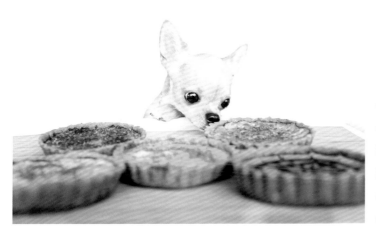

Out of passion to feed more pets out there with organic and natural ingredients found in her fresh, handmade treats, Feed My Paws today has a huge following online in addition to their physical shop.

Pup-friendly tarts above, Yakiniku burger and milk cookies below

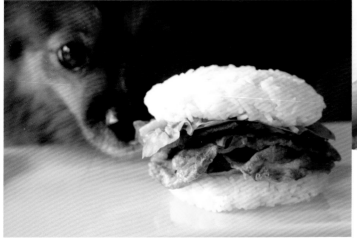

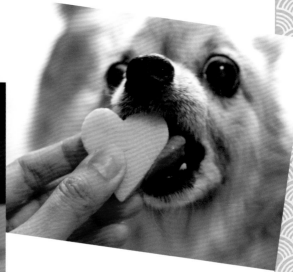

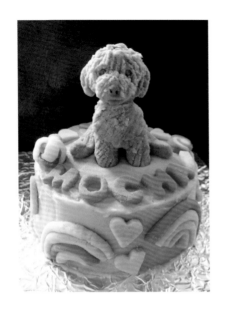

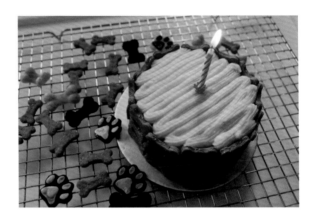

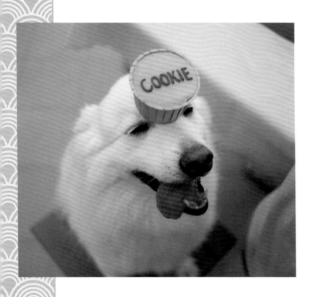

Seeing that many owners like herself would like their pets to be a part of festive occasions and celebrations, Crystle created many festive favorites similar to the ones humans eat so that their pets can have a good feast with their owners during these special times. Her craft not only includes whipping up delicious meals, but she is also talented in recreating life-like edible dog figurines for special occasions. Exotic meat treats like crocodile jerky is also a favorite among her customers, who want only the best for their pets.

Crazy Rich Fact: The Secret Club

When one of the founding fathers of Singapore, Dr. Goh Keng Swee, passed away in 2010, his only son Mr. Goh Kian Chee met reporters at the Pyramid Club in Goodwood Hill, where he spoke of his late father and to thank the public for their kind support. The story published online in 2010 is missing from the archives. That article got many searching for the Pyramid Club, a place almost unheard of by everyone unless you are from the inner circle of Singapore's most elite movers and shakers that shape the country.

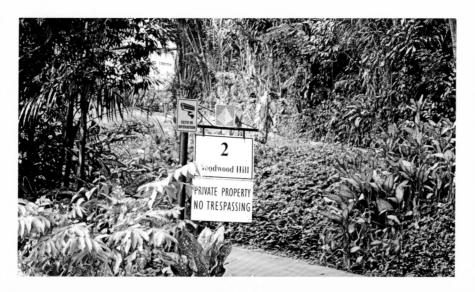

Just a minute away from the hustle and bustle of Orchard Road, Singapore's busiest shopping district and one of the most expensive addresses to have in the country, a small enclave called Goodwood Hill nestled in lush greenery exists quietly at the fringe of the chaos of Orchard Road. On top of the hill boasts one of Singapore's best-kept secrets—an elite club so exclusive that many have not heard of and are unaware of its entire existence.

The Pyramid Club, more than three hundred members strong, is the kind of place Kitty Pong will dream of all day to one day set foot in and be its member but will never come close. A search online for any information on the club, like its location or phone number, will hit a dead wall and all that is published are a few rare archived photos from private events that made its way to the web. A reporter once got hold of the club's number from a government department but after the call was successfully connected, a man from the club's first question was, "How did you get hold of us?" and seemed rather startled to have been discovered. Any form of written questions sent to the club will also go unanswered and silence is how the club hopes any news about it will go away.

Back in 1997, then-Prime Minister of Singapore, Mr. Goh Chok Tong, wanted to throw an important party to recognize the contribution of a group of senior politicians who have for many years been the pillars of the ruling People's Action Party in Parliament. A tribute is needed as they are now required to step down so that new blood can enter to rejuvenate the party. The evening had to be a night to remember and of course, a special venue with great historical significance was needed.

The Pyramid Club was the top choice for the event, picked by the Prime Minister himself. An elegant black and white colonial-era mansion perched on top of Goodwood Hill, it has a sense of arrival just like Tyersall Park, Ah Ma's home in the Crazy Rich Asians series. That evening in May 1997, the local newspaper reported that 140 distinguished guests were treated to some of the finest delicacies for dinner.

The newspaper article in 1997, like the one in 2010, was a very brief mention of the club once in many years. It is a place unknown and unfamiliar to most Singaporeans but is one of the most important and powerful clubs for the top 0.01 percent of the country. The Pyramid is the go-to after-hours club for more than three hundred of the country's most important elites, and it has been said by a non-member that "anyone who is anyone" will be on their list. It is rumored by some to be the location where the real action in Singapore takes place. Politicians, senior military officers, businessmen, and top civil servants congregate here in its well-appointed grounds to forge friendships, exchange news and information, and to mold the country to its best possibility.

Despite the member list of the Pyramid Club reading like a "Who's Who of Singapore," this is not *Tatler*, the country's society magazine for those who want to see and be seen. The fiercely private club goes out of its way to make sure it does not draw attention from the general public. Requests for information from marketing firms that promote and sell memberships for other elite and exclusive clubs across Asia is greeted with plain ignorance. It is simply a place that is unheard of even among people who are sure that they "know it all" when it comes to Singapore's society.

The strict secrecy of the club and its preference to be under the radar only fuels rumors to spread like wildfire. Some well-informed Singaporeans speculate that the club is almost cult-like. It is in reality, however, the club is more like a close-knit fraternity to discuss and execute Singapore's public policy and perhaps much less sensational than the rumors of what this place is like.

Founded in 1963 when Singapore just gained independence from the British and just before the merger with Malaya to form Malaysia, the Pyramid Club came about during one of the most crucial periods in Singapore's road to independence. The club's main purpose, as found written on the Registry of Societies, says, "To provide opportunities and amenities for members [to engage in a] regular exchange of ideas and information on matters of public interest." Its motto: "A pyramid of public service" gives an insight into the main aim of the club. The first president of the club was Dr. Goh Keng Swee, a man so important to Singapore that when he stepped down from politics in 1984, then Prime Minister Mr. Lee Kuan Yew said, "A whole generation of Singaporeans take their present standard of living for granted because you had laid the foundations of the economy of modern Singapore." He was instrumental in setting up the country's Economic Development Board, the Jurong Industrial Estate to draw global multinational corporations to invest in Singapore, and also most importantly GIC (Government of Singapore Investment Corporation), a sovereign wealth fund set up to invest the foreign reserves of Singapore to generate wealth for the country. He was also involved in many other projects to better the lives of Singapore and Singaporeans.

The privacy of the club only falters when the club is used for special occasions and that non-members are invited for an exclusive once-in-a-lifetime visit. Members of the club will never talk publicly about it but the same cannot be said of the visiting non-members. If you ever take the trouble of visiting Goodwood Hill in search of this oasis nestled near the busiest streets of Singapore, look out for a sign that says "PRIVATE PROPERTY, NO TRESPASSING" and also a little logo of the pyramid. You will be disappointed, however, as the thick bushes and well-trimmed trees shroud the entire place in secrecy and there is no glimpse of the building from the main road. Nonetheless, you are steps away from one of Singapore's best-kept secrets, and the best is to let your imagination run wild while at it.

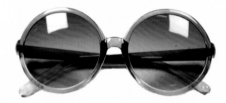

CHAPTER 6:
AMAZING ARCHITECTURE

MARINA BAY SANDS

The most iconic building of the country, Marina Bay Sands is the most Instagrammed hotel in the world thanks to the world's longest infinity pool on the 57th floor. In fact, there are guides online teaching people how to sneak into the famous pool and also people selling themselves just for a chance to have a dip and a photo taken. Nicknamed "ship hotel," "Noah's ark," "ironing board," "surfboard," and the likes, the hotel was completed in 2010 and was the most expensive building in the world at that time, costing USD $5.5 billion.

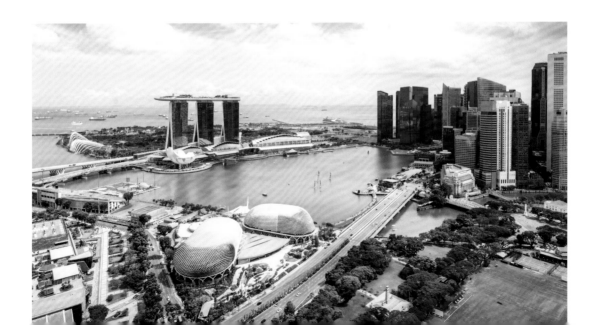

Designed by the world-renowned Moshe Safdie, who in a recent interview called himself a semi-Singaporean, the Israeli architect has designed several iconic buildings in the country. The design of the building was initially inspired by card decks. The owner of the hotel Las Vegas Sands declared the building to be "one of the world's most challenging construction projects and certainly the most expensive stand-alone integrated resort property ever built." The three hotel towers have 2,561 rooms and a continuous lobby at the base to link them. On top of the three buildings is the world's largest public cantilevered platform, featuring a 1,120-foot SkyPark with a capacity of 3,900 people and a 490-foot-long infinity swimming pool.

Marina Bay Sands has proved to be a giant money-making machine for Las Vegas Sands Corp. reaching USD $541 million in the first quarter of 2018. It was announced in 2019 that a fourth tower will be added to the integrated resort and Las Vegas Sands Corp. will spend an approximate USD $3.3 billion on it. The fourth tower will feature about a thousand all-suite hotel rooms, exhibition halls, and a 15,000-seat indoor entertainment arena.

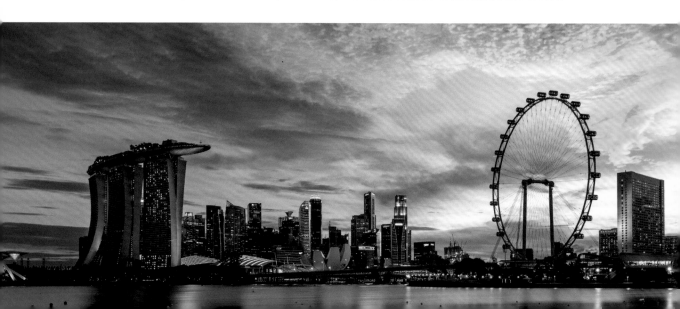

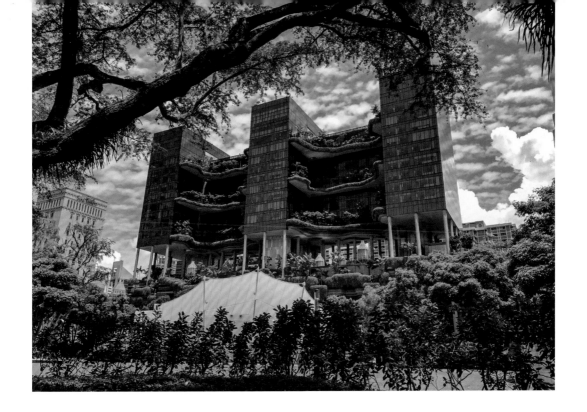

Parkroyal on Pickering

Called a "Hotel in a garden," Parkroyal on Pickering is a unique architectural feat that features 160,000 square feet of terraced gardens that are elevated. The luxury hotel with 367 rooms and suites was designed by WOHA, a Singapore-based architecture firm famous for using extensive greenery in their buildings. The concept of the sky gardens is to be self-sustaining. Through the usage of motion sensors, solar cells, rainwater harvesting, and reclaimed water, they consume minimal energy.

The building has won numerous awards including President's Design of the Year Award in 2013, and Hotel of the Year award from World Architecture News (WAN) Awards.

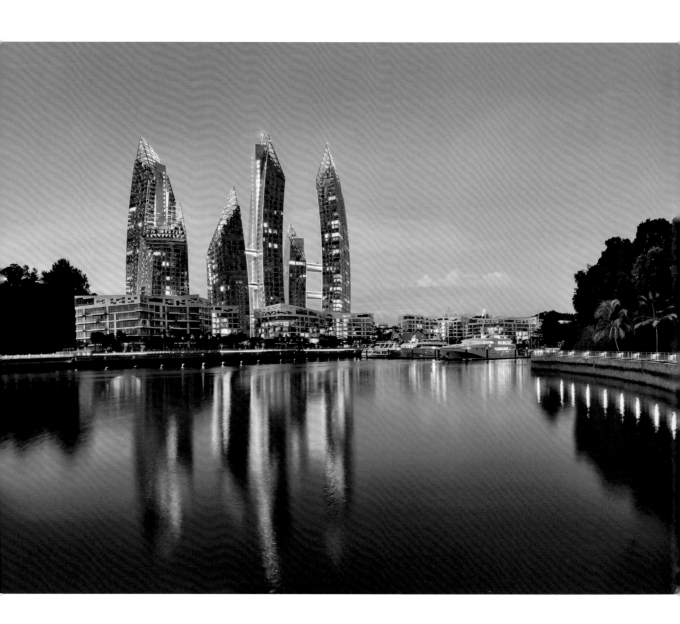

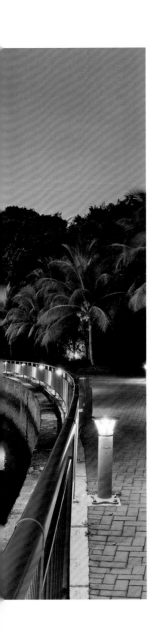

Reflections at Keppel Bay

Designed by the famous Daniel Libeskind, Reflections at Keppel Bay is the most iconic building at the southern waterfront of Singapore by the famous Jewish architect from Poland. Libeskind also won the competition to be the master plan architect for the reconstruction of the World Trade Center in New York.

The luxury waterfront residential complex completed in 2011 has 1,129 units. The property, however, is most famous for the story of a lady who bought eighty-three units of Tower 1A in 2007 for approximately USD $166 million. While returning from a trip to Batam, an Indonesia island forty minutes from Singapore by ferry, Madam Lily Lai, in her fifties, caught sight of the banner advertising the property and decided to take a look. I presume the sales agent that day fell off the chair upon hearing her interest in an entire tower block. The low-profile real estate investor was originally born in Taiwan but is now a Singapore citizen. News of her purchase drew attention when she appealed against her approximately USD $5 million stamp duty bill, arguing that her purchase should be treated as eighty-three separate ones and not as a single contract. She ended up getting a discount of an estimated USD $325,000 following a landmark High Court judgement.

Jewel Changi Airport

The latest attraction in the country and possibly one that will become as famous as the Marina Bay Sands, Jewel Changi Airport, as the name suggest, is one of the best airports in the world. Designed once again by Moshe Safdie, the architect himself says that previously, Changi Airport was known for its world-class service but never for its design. With Jewel, however, the airport now has both. Shaped like a giant nest or donut, the building spans ten floors, five above-ground and five basement levels. The heart of the building is the world's largest indoor waterfall at forty meters tall. the HSBC Rain Vortex is surrounded by lush greeneries and is fast making a layover in Singapore a highly attractive one.

Always a step ahead of others, Jewel was built to improve the competitive position of Singapore's airport against rivals such as Bangkok's Suvarnabhumi International Airport and Kuala Lumpur International Airport. It was built with an intention to combine an urban park and a marketplace. "The component of the traditional mall is combined with the experience of nature, culture, education, and recreation, aiming to provide an uplifting experience. By drawing in both visitors and local residents alike, we aim to create a place where the people of Singapore interact with the people of the world," said Moshe Safdie.

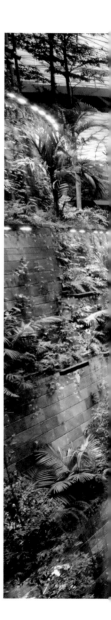

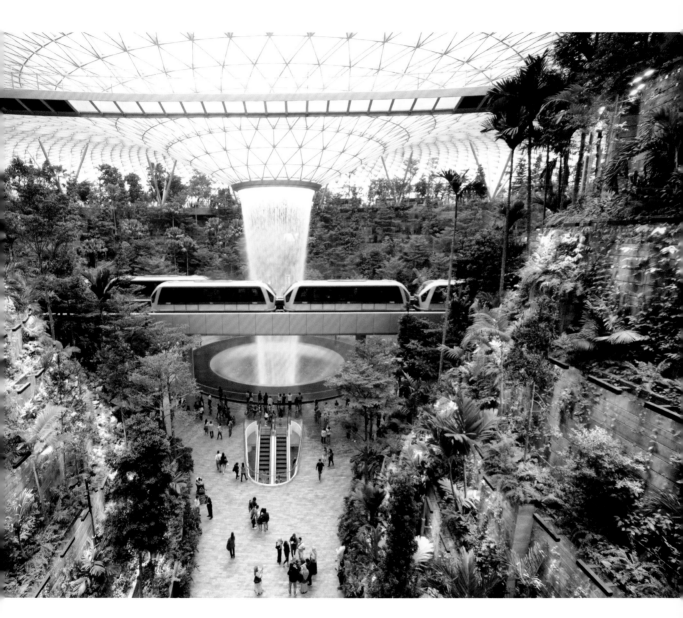

Crazy Rich Fact: Billion-Dollar Building for Prayer

Ever prayed in a billion-dollar building? That's what members of New Creation Church can do every week at the Star in Singapore. Built at an estimated cost of SGD $1 billion (USD $730 million), the Star is composed of the Star Performing Arts Centre owned by the church from level 3 to 11, and the Star Vista, a shopping mall from basement 4 to level 2 owned by CapitaMalls Asia.

New Creation Church proudly announced in 2016 that its 5,000-seat Star Performing Arts Centre built at a cost of an estimated USD $367 million was fully paid for after it had been used for church services since 2012. Known for its ability to raise record amount of money in a day due to its ultra-rich congregation, the church made headlines in 2010 when it managed to raise USD $15.5 million in a day. It broke its previous record of raising USD $13.81 million in a day in 2009 and also the 2008 record of raising USD $13.23 million in a day.

Rock Production, the business arm of the church, purchased the land on a sixty-year lease for approximately USD $138 million. The shopping mall component of the development cost about USD $350 million.

The independent church was started in 1983 in a public flat with just 25 people attending its Sunday Service before it exploded to its current figures of about 33,000 Sunday attendees (as of 2019).

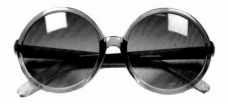

ACKNOWLEDGMENTS

First of all, I would like to thank my dear friend Dawn Yang for sharing with me the first chapter of *Crazy Rich Asians* on a random afternoon during brunch in 2014. It led me to being completely obsessed with the series, being crazy enough to create a tour to meet fellow fans, and finally, writing this book.

I would also like to thank these amazing people for helping with the book: Rachel Sia, Ng Po Loong, Kelly Chen, Ming Tan, and Crystle Tan.

Lastly, a big thank you to Kevin Kwan for his amazing series that took all of us fans on such a wild ride. Thank you for bringing Singapore to the world and making us cool so effortlessly. Thank you for writing a book that has so many things that only Singaporeans will understand (like Bishop See Bei Sien's name). Thank you for letting our future generations have literature about Singapore that is a global hit and yet so familiar. They can grow up reading about Lau Pa Sat while being inside Lau Pa Sat, book in one hand, satay in another. You are our national treasure.